THE RECIPE FOR LIFE

Sally Bee

THE RECIPE FOR LIFE

Sally Bee

Healthy eating for real people

Collins

dedication

This book is dedicated to all my very precious and gorgeous friends. You know who you are.

But especially, this is for Dogan, the love of my life. Always.

First published in 2011 by Collins
an imprint of HarperCollins*Publishers*
77–85 Fulham Palace Road
London W6 8JB

www.harpercollins.co.uk

10 9 8 7 6 5 4 3 2 1

Photography © Myles New 2011
Text © Sally Bee 2011

Publishing Director: Jenny Heller
Editorial: Helen Hawksfield and Lizzy Gray

Sally Bee asserts her moral right to be identified as the author of this work.

A catalogue record for this book is available from the British Library.

ISBN: 978-0-00-734407-9

Colour reproduction, printing and binding by L.e.g.o. S.p.a., Italy

contents

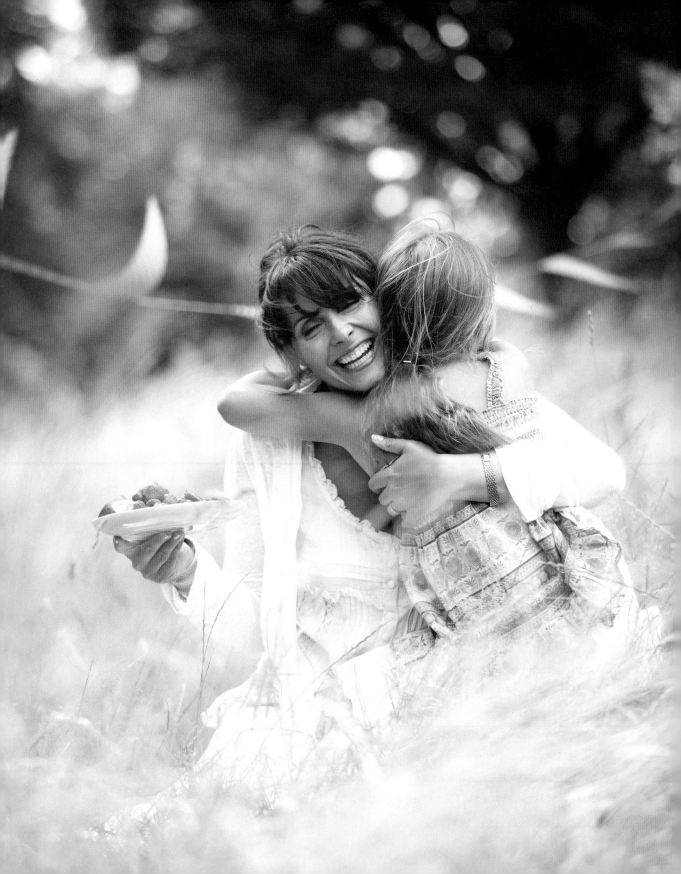

introduction

In my first book, *The Secret Ingredient*, apart from all the lovely, healthy recipes, I wrote about my experiences when I suffered three heart attacks in the space of one week at the tender age of 36. I spoke about the moment my husband was told to come and say his goodbyes, and about the immediate effects the experience had on both my family and myself. The trauma I suffered was huge, both physically and emotionally, and it took such a long time to recover to the level of fitness that I have now, happily, achieved.

So, moving on, I'd now like to share with you the next stage of my recovery, which will lead on nicely to the delicious recipes included in this book. It may seem like a strange partnership: survival, recovery and food. But if you read on, I think you'll start to understand what good healthy food has meant to me, and maybe it will help you understand your relationship with food a little better. I hope so…

my fragile heart

To briefly recap on my story so far, I suffered from three very serious heart attacks when I was aged just 36. At the time I was mum to a five-year-old, a two-year-old and my baby was just nine months old. So life was pretty busy, as you can imagine. My heart attacks hit me completely out of the blue. I was, or thought I was, fit and strong and healthy. As a mum of three young children, there was never time to sit back and be poorly, but I was happy. My heart attacks weren't caused by the usual heart disease, rather, a rare and usually fatal condition called Spontaneous Coronary Artery Dissection (SCAD). In essence, what happened was that the main artery inside my heart that was responsible for feeding the large bulk of the heart muscle with blood and oxygen fell apart, or 'dissected'. If my artery had just dissected in a small area, the doctors could have performed a bypass operation to save me, but because the dissection went from the top of the artery to the very bottom, the doctors knew there was nothing they could do to save me, so they simply left me alone and told my husband to come in and say goodbye.

Just as my husband Dogan came into the operating room, and I realised that I was still alive, my battle began. The next few minutes were dramatic. My body was giving up but my mind had taken control. I had allowed myself to think about the children … and my life … and I wasn't ready to give it all up yet. It was a struggle because by this stage my failing heart and other organs had other ideas – good job I'm a strong-minded chick!

The following days passed in a bit of a blur. I couldn't move, talk, cough or cry without my heart going into melt down. The nursing staff where struggling to understand what was happening to me. The monitor that I was constantly hooked up to couldn't recognise the rhythms that my heart was getting into, yet it kept coming out of all the little episodes, still ticking! After a few days, I demanded that they wash my hair. I was told in no uncertain terms that I had no chance. I couldn't even get up to go to the bathroom at this stage, so a hair wash was completely out of the question. Let's just say I have great powers of persuasion, and with a team of doctors and nurses on stand-by 'just in case', I was shuffled on my back to the end of my bed, with my head just tipping off the end and my hair was washed. It felt amazing. When my mum arrived bearing my lipstick the following day, I knew I had to continue with this approach to have any chance of a normal life again.

But it wasn't so easy. Between writing my previous book and this one, my lovely mum was diagnosed with cancer and, just a short nine months later, she died. The grief and sadness we all suffered when we learned about her diagnosis was at times unbearable and overwhelming, but at least we knew what to expect, so could begin to prepare ourselves. We knew that mum's journey from this point had a beginning, a middle and an end. I remember very vividly the day she was told it was terminal. We all had a big cry and a little quiet time, then arranged a big, happy party for all our family and friends the following weekend. Looking back now, how crazy that seems. Mum spent the final two weeks of her life in a wonderful hospice near my home and my dad and I spent every possible moment with her. Those two weeks were the most precious weeks of my life. Although unbearably painful, we all knew and understood what was going to happen and my mum accepted it fully, I think. This didn't make it any less upsetting or painful, but it did mean that we knew what we had to do. My mum even managed to make her own funeral arrangements, being bossy about what we were allowed to sing, wear and eat!

In contrast, after my heart attacks, I didn't know what I was supposed to do. I hadn't been told I would definitely die but I also wasn't told that I would definitely live. Because my heart condition is so very rare, my cardiologists couldn't find any other survivors that I could talk to. So I was sent home without any positive prognosis, just a continuing feeling of impending doom and uncertainty. I was scared of everything in the beginning. Absolutely everything. I was afraid to laugh, afraid to cry, to get angry or upset, afraid to shout and love. I was so scared to move too quickly, I couldn't drive, I couldn't play with my children or go out with my friends. I was afraid to go out of my front door and, at the same time, afraid to stay at home. I couldn't seem to find a way out of the prison that was now my life.

Although my family and friends were happy and pleased to see me back home, they didn't really understand what I was going through. I don't think I helped the situation, as I was a great pretender! When I got a little stronger, but was still struggling to cope with day-to-day things, I would go through a great long process to appear normal to those around me. My eldest son was five years old at this time and he was desperate for me to pick him up from school, just like the other mums, but I couldn't manage the walk around the block to walk him home as he wanted. So instead, I would spend the entire day getting ready. Washing and drying my hair was a three-hour process, including all the rests I needed in between. Then I would get my mum or husband to drive me round the corner to school, long before any of the other parents arrived. I could sit quietly on the bench in the playground to get my breath back. When the other parents arrived I would smile happily and give everyone a big wave. I could see them wondering what all the fuss was about. They had heard that I was gravely ill, yet here I was looking fine! If only they knew. So my super little chap would run out of school and I would be able to stand up and throw my arms around him and hear all his excitable babble from his day that just had to come out the moment he saw me. Mission accomplished. I was a normal mum for my five-year-old precious boy. I would then sit down while a friend walked Tarik home, and when everyone else left the playground I would be quietly helped back to the car and be driven home. Exhausted.

So life continued like this for a while and I suppose for that time I accepted that this was as good as it was going to get. Then I was lucky enough to reach a tipping point, which changed my life again, forever. I had just reached the first-year anniversary of my heart attacks and was due at one of my regular check-ups with my cardiologist. He told me that I needed to have a special scan to detect a possible problem in my aorta. (Because my main heart artery had dissected from top to bottom, it was thought that this dissection might have started above, in my aorta, causing a life-threatening aneurism.) This was a potential problem all along apparently, but as nobody imagined I would survive a year, it seemed unnecessary to worry me further. But as I had reached this point, there was a strange urgency to deal with the problem. They were going to pull a team together to perform the scan in three weeks time and, if they found the aneurism, I would have two choices: either live with it until it killed me, or operate, without great chances of survival. Not the best choices in the world. I felt like I'd been given another date that I might die. During the three weeks leading up to my scan, I was incredibly agitated and felt I had to keep myself busy. When I wasn't crying, I was making arrangements, again, 'just in case'. I got all the children's clothes organised for the following season and gave my girlfriends instructions on where to buy their clothes

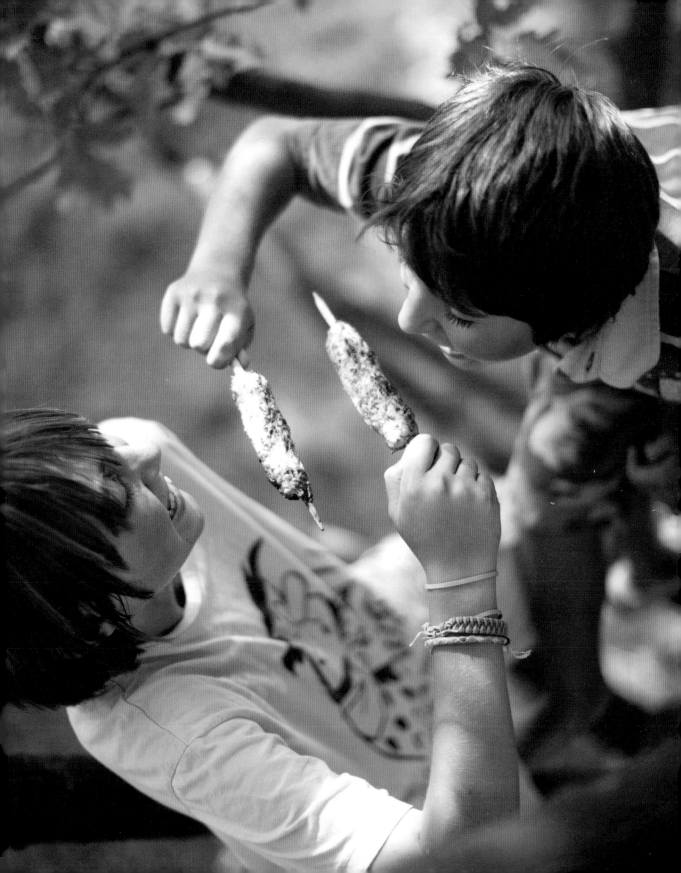

if I wasn't around. I taught Dogan how to plait my daughter's hair, how to measure out the children's medicine and sign up at school for parents' evening appointments. I spoke to his friends and told them not to let him turn to the bottle if anything happened to me – and he wasn't allowed to get involved with any big-boobed blondes who weren't right for my children! Dark days passed. The day of my scan dawned and, for the first time in three weeks, I was calm – just like the weather. You see the night before I had realised something that blew my mind. I realised that I had got myself into such a state that I was more afraid of living than I was of dying.

All this time I had been looking back and not forwards. I had been trying to come to terms with what had happened to me and was just surviving, not living. Now I was facing the day that my life might end and, it sounds crazy, but it was almost a relief. I suddenly realised that I just couldn't do this any more. I couldn't continue to live with this constant fear. I didn't want to live if I was afraid of life. I wasn't being the mummy I wanted to be to my children, I certainly wasn't the wife that my husband had chosen to spend the rest of his life with. Death didn't seem as scary as a life of fear at this point.

I thought long and hard about my life, or lack of it, and then thought back to the Sally who had demanded her hair got washed while being cared for in a high-dependency unit, and the Sally who made sure she had lipstick on even when she was on the critical list. I felt my blood run cold and my goosebumps jump. OK, if today was the day my life ended, then so be it. Bring it on! I was ready. If I had to die today, then that was my fate. But if there was any chance that I didn't have this horrible problem in my aorta, then look out world because I was going to get back up and kick its ass! I had suffered a fright, many people do, but I was lucky that I was still here and still breathing. At that moment I made a pact with myself that, if I could get through today, I was going to start living again. But this life had to be one without fear – or I wasn't interested. I allowed myself to imagine for a moment for that I had a future. I looked forwards and imagined that I did survive another ten, twenty, thirty or even forty years. And do you know what the most frightening part of that daydream was? The scariest part of my future was not living with the fear of dying but living while being afraid to live.

You may have gathered, simply by the fact that I am able to write this book, that I didn't have an aneurism in my aorta. The news came back that half my heart muscle was damaged and in failure, but the other half was somehow miraculously compensating. The doctors still couldn't tell me that I'd be OK, but that didn't matter any more because I now believed that I had a future and the quality of it was in my hands. I was back in the driving seat. It was still scary, if I'm honest, especially for my family, but it was my life and I wasn't going to waste another moment.

choosing life

So moving along five years, I'm still out there living my life and enjoying every minute. I'm as energetic as I can be, some days more than others. I still have to rest and take good care of myself all the time but this has become normal and I think I absorb it pretty well now. I am on an aggressive drug regime (and will be for the rest of my life), which, in turn, can affect my kidneys and liver but, so far, my body is coping really well with everything I throw at it. I can get some accusing looks sometimes when I bounce out of my car all colourful and glowy and put my blue disabled badge in the window. I sometimes feel that people would be happier if they saw me limping to be worthy of my blue badge – but the reality is, I must never put myself in a position where I am lifting heavy objects, including shopping, or struggling a distance if I am suffering from fatigue. So my blue badge is a must, as I would never want to put myself in a dangerous position, especially for the sake of a couple of shopping bags!

My cardiologists are still happily amazed with my progress and, considering the damage my heart has suffered, my power output is fantastic. They cannot explain why I have recovered so well. I can I put everything down to the food that I eat and the way that I move.

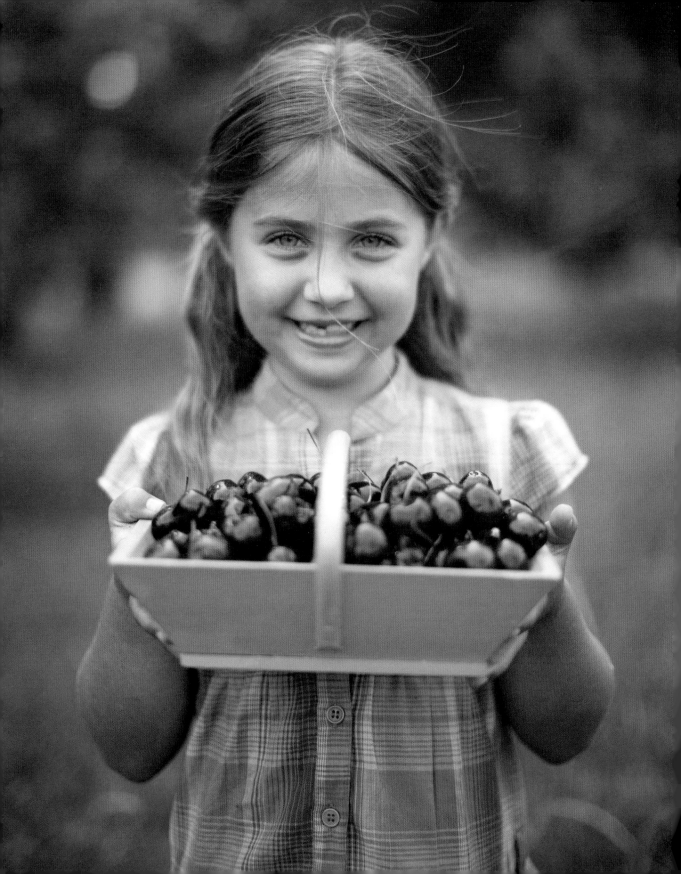

a healthy lifestyle – your best insurance policy

So how can my experience help you? Well, whether you are a heart patient or not, the truth is that these days, generally, our diets and lifestyles are not helpful in maintaining a healthy heart. My heart attacks were caused by a very rare condition, which none of you should have to worry about, but the results are the same as for anyone who has suffered a heart event: compromised heart health; ongoing medication; and the need and desire to maintain good health for as long as possible into the future. I am not a trained medical nutritionist so I would recommend that, if you have any health issues or concerns, you make an appointment with your GP who will be able to direct you to the correct information for your particular condition. If you are lucky enough to be in good health just now, it is vitally important not to waste your opportunity of securing ongoing good health for your future. You are coming from a great starting point but still, you must not underestimate the potential for problems.

We eat for enjoyment but the No. 1 reason we eat is to nourish ourselves and take care of ourselves … let's do it well.

I survived my heart attacks because I had a good insurance policy – not financial but physical. Beforehand I had taken regular exercise, I had eaten a healthy diet, I didn't smoke, drink or take drugs. And living a healthy lifestyle is not only good for your heart, it will help guard against other diseases, including some cancers and, as if that wasn't benefit enough, living a healthy lifestyle will make you feel happier and look younger, too.

I have to let you into a little secret here. This book is not only for those of you who have a health issue or are recovering from poor health. We all deserve a treat and a pamper, and actually caring about our looks shows that we are looking after our health, too. After my heart attacks I was obviously devastated and have written about how desperate I felt at times. Well, I can also share with you that I shed almost as many tears over the fact that I lost a lot of my hair! I think it was probably due to the shock and the medication that I was on, but my cardiologist didn't have it on his list of priorities to deal with. I did! I found it devastating – thank heavens for the magic of hair extensions. It may seem a little frivolous or superficial, but actually, our looks can have a massive impact on the way that we feel. So if you feel that you'd like to regain a little of your youthful complexion or shiny hair as well as the energy of a 21-year-old (I wish!), then try eating a nourishing and healthy diet and you will soon start to notice some wonderfully superficial beauty bonuses. Whether you are a strong and energetic teenager, a busy young mum or dad or a grandparent taking life easy, I hope that my recipes will entice you to lead the healthiest possible lifestyle for you.

my philosophy

My philosophy about food is very simple. It is the only thing that can give us our health. Other things can take it away, such as drinking, smoking and a lazy lifestyle. But food is what makes us what we are. The food we eat affects our energy levels and our sleep patterns. It affects how happy we feel and the way we look – our hair and our skin

I hope my recipes prove that you don't have to eat lettuce and jacket potatoes all day to have a nutritious dinner, and you don't have to obsess over calories to maintain weight loss.

I am living proof that eating a rounded, healthy diet works. I was, quite literally, at death's door and now I'm probably more energetic than many of my friends. I feel the effects of a poor diet within minutes. If I'm away from home for a few days and can't eat what my body needs, I very quickly begin to feel tired and lethargic and fed up! I can't make you any promises about your personal health, but you can rest assured that the healthy ingredients that I choose are all thought to be health giving in some way by doctors and scientists who are properly trained to comment.

So all my recipes will offer you nutrition and are quick and easy to make. You don't have to be an expert chef to give yourself and your family good health – you may just need a few new ideas and a gentle nudge in the right direction.

If you've just been diagnosed with heart disease or another health problem, don't think that this is a prison sentence and don't assume that 'diet' food is your only choice. Try to see your situation in a positive light. You have a fantastic opportunity to take control of your future health. You have the chance to make some wonderfully positive changes that will not only benefit you but the family and friends around you. There are a few tips that I can give you from my experiences that might help you to get on the right track to a healthier future:

* Learn to listen to your body after you've eaten. Which foods lift your mood and help you to feel energised? Which food makes you sleepy, lethargic or sad? I think that when you listen well, you'll soon realise that natural, unprocessed foods will lift you and energise you rather than tire you out. But don't take my word for it – try it for yourself.

* Take notice of how you move and start to push yourself a little. When you are walking around the shops or to and from work, ask yourself if you could walk a little quicker. Then see how you feel when you do speed up for a while. Look in the mirror – you'll probably see a lovely flushed face smiling back at you. Very healthy!

* If this is all new to you, make a commitment to have a healthy week. Spend the week eating good food and incorporating a little more movement (otherwise known as exercise) into your routine, and then properly listen to your body at the end of that week. Have you felt more energised? Have you slept well? Are you ready for another, even better and healthier week?

* Set some goals that you'd like to achieve. Maybe it's a change of job, or looking good for a wedding in the summer or trying for a baby or running a marathon. Whatever it is that you'd like to achieve, by taking control of your health through nutrition, you should feel proud and capable of improving your self-discipline and motivation in all areas of your life. Taking control of your diet is just the beginning…

The thing that surprises people when they start to change the way they view food and exercise in the right way is that it isn't a chore and they don't feel that they are depriving themselves. I know that if you follow some of my recipes and start to eat for nourishment (and enjoyment of course!), you will feel and see the benefits on the inside and the outside. And what

I hope will happen is that you won't want to go back to your unhealthy ways, because you'll love the feeling of wellbeing too much to let it slip.

the missing piece of the puzzle

After my heart attacks, my body was badly damaged and was struggling to survive and I had to find a way to help fix it. This certainly wasn't going to be helped purely by low-calorie snacks, soups and drinks without any nutritional benefit, and being slim alone wouldn't fix the problem. Therefore I needed to make sure that every mouthful of food I ate gave my body some nutritional value. And at the same time, I had three young children at home and it was important to me that they grew up with a good healthy attitude towards food, just as I had done. I didn't want them to think that a diet of mung beans and spinach was normal. Our meal times at home were, and forever will be, precious times. Meal times offer an emotional outlet for the day's events. It's a time when we share our stories and concerns and funny moments. And to match this mood, it's crucial that the meals we eat feed our heart, our body and our soul. Our food is not just required to stop us from feeling hungry. It is also not just needed to give our body nutrition, although that's obviously a most important part; food has to satisfy our emotions as well as our hunger. This is the missing piece of the puzzle that you may have been struggling to find. It's also necessary for our food to feed our emotions. Imagine if you sat down every day to a green salad and jacket potato because you were on a 'diet'. I think life would be pretty miserable and unsatisfying. Maybe that's why dieters run for a big chunk of chocolate at the drop of a hat. Maybe it's not the calories or the sugar that they crave, maybe it's the emotional fulfilment they are lacking.

Food has to satisfy our emotions as well as our hunger. This is the missing piece of the puzzle that you may have been struggling to find.

portion distortion

In today's 'the-more-you-get-the-better' society, package sizes keep growing. Giant bottles of cola, extra large bags of crisps and king-size chocolate bars are all the rage. But as these foods get larger, so do our waistlines. Bigger packages and food items apparently distort portion control.

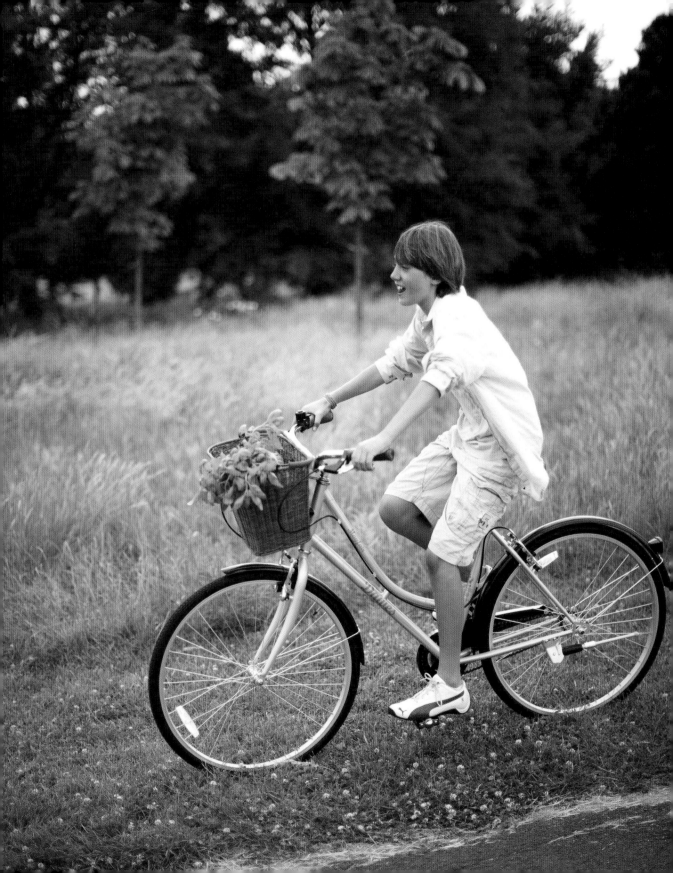

Having said this, I actually struggle with the notion that you should only eat a certain 'size' of meal. Instead, I would prefer you to listen to your body and know when you've had enough. A large nutritious, balanced meal will do you more good than a small portion of processed food. It's also really important to take into consideration what you eat over a whole day, not just at one meal … and how much you move. If I am having a busy day with the children, running around all day long, I can get really hungry and eat a larger portion of food than usual. But as long as my intake and output are matched, I'm in good shape. Obviously, if I'm having a calmer day, maybe sitting at my computer writing, then my output is lower, so my intake needs to be lower. It's not rocket science and you don't have to be an expert to work it out – but you do need to get in tune with your body and work out if you are eating because you're hungry, or for some other reason. Having said all of that, if you are overweight and would like to lose some weight, do make an effort to cut your portion sizes across the board. Using a smaller plate is always a good starting point, and always try to have your vegetable portion larger than your meat or carbohydrate portion. Good luck – you can do it!

too busy to exercise?

Me too! However, it's crucially important that we all exercise. My future health depends on it, and so does yours.

I think it's wonderful if you enjoy going to the gym, running races or swimming across lakes, but many people don't want to do that … or can't do that! However, that is still no excuse. Another word for exercise is movement, and we can all do that in one way or another. I am far too busy to stop my life to go to the gym, but I have time to go for a bike ride with the children or quickly take the dog for a walk. When I go to do my supermarket shopping, I'll try to do a 60-minute trip to the isles in 40 minutes. That gets my heart rate up – and the fridge gets filled at the same time. Perfect.

I read a study once that showed how some scientists had changed the way that a group did ten daily activities every day. So instead of buying ready-prepared vegetables, they peeled and chopped them, and instead of using the TV remote, they got up to change the channel. They used stairs instead of escalators and walked around the office when they were on the telephone at work instead of sitting down to talk. These sound like pretty, simple, gentle changes. However, the shocking results showed that the people who took part in the study had, at the end of a one month trial, done the equivalent of an 120 mile walk over the space of that month. Simply by changing the way they did ten domestic things a day. What are you going to change? Remember, small steps make a big difference.

You'll notice that most of my recipes have only short instructions and are very uncomplicated. That's because I believe in making life as easy as possible and just don't have time to spend hours preparing food. If it takes longer to cook than it does to eat, I've failed! An hour sitting over dinner, chatting to my family is a joy. An hour standing preparing food is a chore.

you're not alone!

Staying healthy through nutrition is such an important thing to do. If you struggle sometimes to stay motivated, remember you are not alone and it might help you to join forces with other people who are also trying to maintain great health. Maybe get a few friends together once a week to share experiences and recipes. Don't be afraid to set up a walking group – you'll probably be amazed at the response – we all need a friend sometimes and we all enjoy the company of others so people will probably thank you for being the one to get everyone else organised. If you enjoy the internet, there are countless forums where you can chat to other people about improving lifestyle, swapping stories and experiences and, by all means, please feel free to write to me. I love to hear other people's stories and still look for inspiration and motivation myself. It's lovely to encourage each other, it's liberating to achieve great results and it's rewarding and fulfilling to pass our successes on to others. Enjoy your healthy future, enjoy your mealtimes with family and friends and feel proud that you have decided to make some effective (and delicious) changes to your nourishment that will, I hope, prove to be your insurance policy for the future.

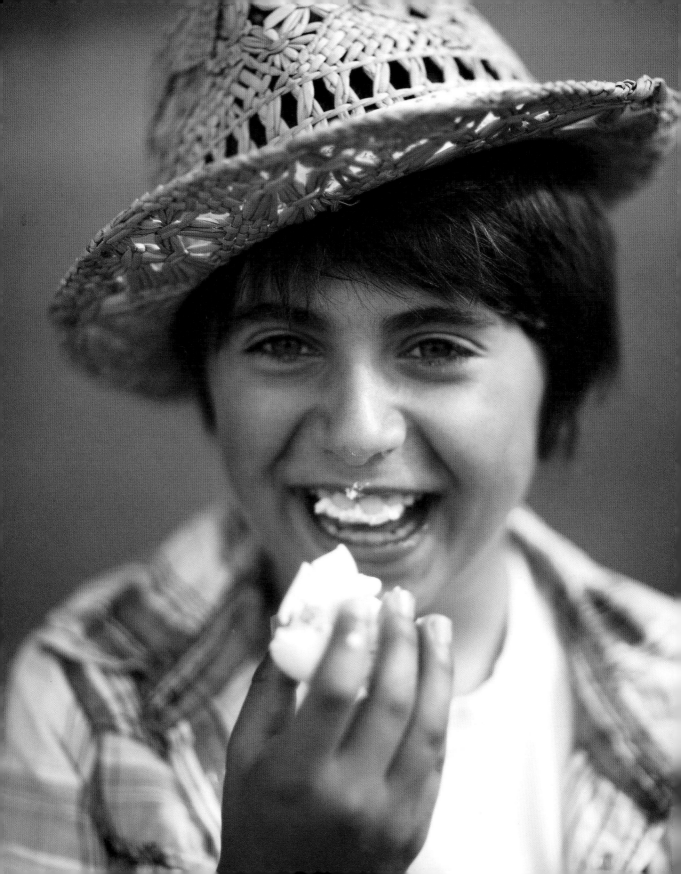

making changes in the kitchen

One of the most important messages I want to stress is that you should not feel intimidated by science, experts or chefs. If you feel you are ready to make some changes to the way you eat and would like to be healthier through food, I want you to know that you can easily do it. It's not rocket science, you won't have to start eating foods that you can't pronounce and can't find in the shops and you do not need to deprive yourself, feel hungry or bullied by anyone!

It's all very well knowing the principles of healthy eating. I think that most of us know that, in order to eat a healthy diet, we need to cut down on fat, sugar and salt and eat more fresh fruit and vegetables and, if we eat meat, we need to try to eat more chicken and fish than red meat. But knowing how to translate that knowledge into a plate of food at the end of a busy day that is healthy, quick and easy to make, affordable, tasty and enticing to the whole family is quite a tall order! But totally possible. Just take a moment to flick through this book and look at the lovely pictures of the dishes. Do they look like the kind of food you eat when you're on a diet? Absolutely not! Yes, every dish in this book is low on the fat, sugar and salt. Sure, many of the recipes contain olive oil, but in small and healthy amounts.

You'll notice that most of my recipes have only short instructions and are very uncomplicated. That's because I believe in making life as easy as possible and just don't have time to spend hours preparing food. If it takes longer to cook than it does to eat, I've failed! An hour sitting over dinner chatting to my family is a joy. An hour standing preparing food is a chore.

my super superfoods

I love pretty much all veggies, chicken and fish – but below is a list of my tip-top superfoods that I couldn't live without. I recommend that you incorporate these into your diet on a regular basis.

* Onions, garlic and olive oil. You'll see that most of my savoury dishes include onions, garlic and olive oil. This is because, besides being a

great base for most dishes, these ingredients are proven to have special health-giving properties, especially when heated together. Onions and garlic belong to the same family and both have a protective action on the circulatory system. Together, they also work as a diuretic and have an antibiotic action. These three ingredients are also proven to help lower blood cholesterol. So, as long as you and your partner go for the garlic, everybody's happy!

* Sweet potatoes. So many of our staple dishes contain potatoes. Now I am a massive fan of the spud, and like to promote its health benefits regularly – but problems can arise when we add butter or fat to improve its taste. In comparison, the sweet potato is very moist and doesn't need anything adding to improve the taste or texture. In fact, sweet potatoes contain everything you need all in one tidy little parcel. Sweet potatoes are a great source of vitamin E because they are fat free. They are also a great source of fibre, betacarotene and vitamins A and C, and are wonderful for a low-carb diet.

* Tomatoes. Tomatoes are packed with potassium and vitamins and are wonderfully low in calories. Eat them cooked or raw, it really doesn't matter – just eat them! Tomatoes are a superfood that gives great nutrition whichever way you look at it. Raw tomatoes are a good source of vitamin C and are high in vitamin A. Cooked tomatoes provide lycopene, an antioxidant thought to reduce cancer risk and cardiovascular disease. Lycopene is especially well absorbed into the body when the tomatoes are cooked and have a little olive oil added – think chilli and spaghetti sauce and, actually, most of the sauce-based dishes throughout this book! Kids don't like tomatoes? Don't give them straight from the refrigerator – they are much nicer at room temperature. Try lovely sweet cherry tomatoes just off the windowsill. Delicious!

* Fish. Oily fish, such as mackerel, salmon, sardines and trout are a rich source of omega-3. Omega-3 is proven to help against heart disease.

* Nuts and seeds. The oils in nuts and seeds, especially almonds, walnuts and peanuts, may help protect against heart disease and possibly some

cancers, too. They are high in fat, but it's the type of fat that is essential as part of a healthy diet, and are great when lightly sprinkled on salads or as a crunchy topping for bakes.

* Green tea. Green tea is believed to protect against heart disease and some cancers. The antioxidants in green tea have been shown to be powerful. Since ancient times, green tea has been considered by the proponents of traditional Chinese medicine as a healthy beverage.

* Berries. Red and blue berries such as raspberries, blueberries and redcurrants contain vitamin C and other antioxidants and are lovely and tasty in desserts or salads.

* Salad leaves. Dark green leafy vegetables are a great source of iron, which helps keep your blood in healthy condition. Add a pile of dark green leaves to your meal as often as you can.

* Spinach. I like to add some raw spinach to many of my salads. It's rich in vitamin C, calcium and betacarotene. It boosts folic acid levels and helps to keep bones and blood healthy. If it's good enough for Popeye, it's good enough for me! Spinach needs to be eaten with vitamin C to ensure optimum absorption, so either add some orange segments to your salad or have a drink of fresh orange juice with your meal.

* Carrots. Bugs Bunny loves them, they're incredibly versatile and they're available all year round at your local grocery shop. Carrots are chock-full of betacarotene, which the body converts to vitamin A for a slew of benefits, including maintenance of healthy teeth and bones, regulation of the immune system and protection from infections. Vitamin A also plays an important role in maintaining normal vision and preventing blindness, lending some truth to the old adage about carrots being good for your eyes. Carrots are rich in potassium, a good source of vitamin C and a great source of vitamin A, as well as fibre.

* Water. Yes, you heard it right – water is one of my superfoods. We all need to drink far more water than we do. Try to aim for eight glasses a

day. Being dehydrated can cause headaches and tiredness and it's easy to confuse thirst for hunger. Before you sit down to a big meal or reach for the snacks, have a glass of water, just to see if that's what your body is really craving.

calories are our friends

In my previous book, I spoke about the fact that I don't like to count calories. Instead, I prefer to use good, natural ingredients and know that my meals are offering a true health benefit. A low-calorie meal doesn't necessarily mean a nutritious meal. Of course it's important to keep the fat content low and you'll notice that all my recipes are low on fat, sugar and salt, but what is most important is that the ingredients offer you a health benefit. You will feel better for eating well. So I just want to re-emphasise that point to you. Calories are actually good for us as long as they come in the right form. We need calories to give us energy, which allows us to exercise and, of course, we get a great health benefit from that. Don't ever waste calories on sweet fizzy drinks and try not to fill up on cakes, biscuits and crisps because these will, of course, add on weight without any health benefit whatsoever. But do feel free to eat a good portion of a healthy, balanced meal and, if you do it right, snacking will become a thing of the past anyway.

make substitutions

If you are taking a look at some of your other cookbooks and fancy doing a favourite recipe, remember to look at it through your healthy glasses! Go with the recipe but don't feel afraid to make substitutions. There are many sensible substitutions that you can make, either when cooking my recipes or anyone else's. Any white fish can be substituted for any other white fish, and any meat for your preferred meat. For example, a chilli dish using red meat can easily be made using turkey mince, which is very low in fat. Vegetables can be easily swapped to suit your taste buds or what you have left in the refrigerator – just try to keep the textures similar.

However, there are a few golden rules of substituting when making a favourite recipe more healthy.

* Butter. A recipe will often call for butter in a sauce and this is often only included to make it shine. Try the same recipe, but leave the butter out or try to substitute a small amount of olive oil instead. This probably won't work for a sweet dish, but it may do the trick for a savoury one. I'll bet it is still as good.

* Salt. Avoid adding salt 99.9 per cent of the time! I have only added a little celery salt into a couple of my recipes and that's because they just absolutely need it. However, the rest of the time I substitute lemon juice for the salt. It gives the same sharp bite without the bad health risks. Get rid of your salt mill off the dinner table and always have lemon wedges to hand instead. You'll be surprised how quickly you'll forget you ever used salt.

* Mayonnaise. If you are following a salad recipe that uses mayo, substitute some low-fat crème fraîche or low-fat fromage frais and mix them with a little lemon juice.

* Buttery mashed potato. If a recipe is telling you to serve an otherwise healthy dish with buttery mashed potato, don't ruin all your good work. Instead, try mashed sweet potato, which doesn't need any butter to mash it up, or serve the dish with brown rice or nutritious new potatoes. If you absolutely love buttery mashed potato, go for it in a small portion on special occasions. Life is too short to not have a treat every now and then!

* Ice cream. The perfect substitution for ice cream is low-fat yogurt. There are so many varieties to choose from and many are now no-fat. Crème fraîche, thick Greek yogurt or bio-yogurt – try them all and see which you like the best. Try freezing them for added excitement at pudding time!

* Tortilla wraps. This sounds like a strange one – but be aware of so called 'healthy' recipes that use flour tortilla wraps. The shop-bought wraps are all very high in fat, and often use hydrogenated fats which are a complete no-no! Try using iceberg lettuce leaves to wrap your ingredients up instead, or wholemeal pitta bread is another great substitution.

* Salads. Salads are, in my opinion, most definitely misunderstood! People sometimes feel a little sad and depressed if they order a salad at a restaurant – feeling maybe quietly pleased that they are sticking to a so called 'diet', but their heart will be aching for a real meal and a treat. Well, you'll be pleased to know that my salads, while being packed with goodness, are so far from the bad old days of limp lettuce and soggy tomato. I love salads that are filling and satisfying. Salads can be served warm or cold, light as a side dish and meatier as a main course. My salad dressings are based on olive oil and lemon juice but there are so many flavours you can add to this combination – mustard, vinegar, chilli, herbs and spices. Don't be afraid to experiment. If there is an ingredient you don't like, swap it for something you do … but don't be afraid to try something new!

So, I now hand over to you. Buy fresh ingredients, take a little time to plan ahead and enjoy delicious, nutritious food that will help you feel energised and healthy. Remember, if I can do it – you can do it!

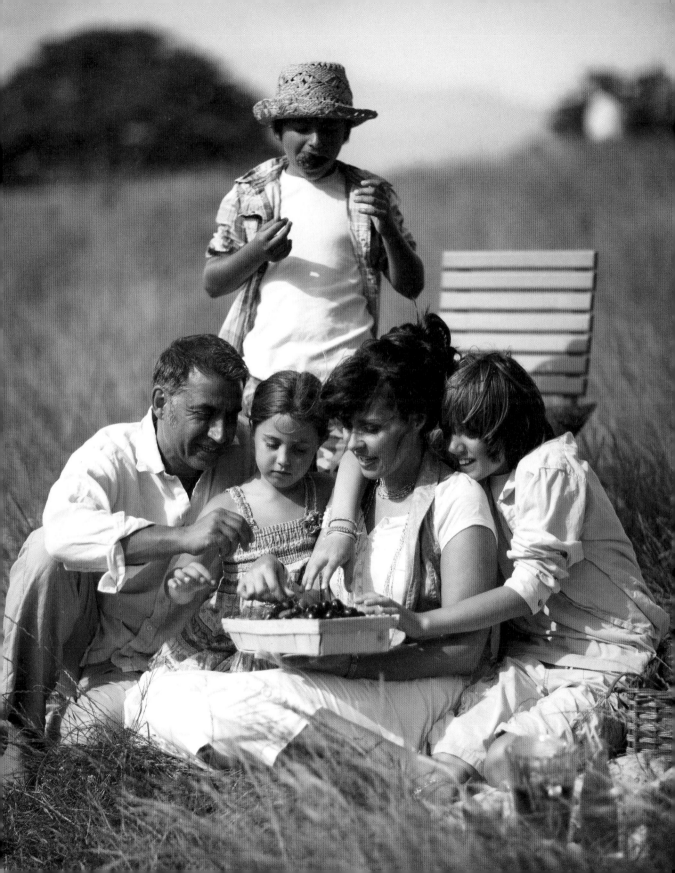

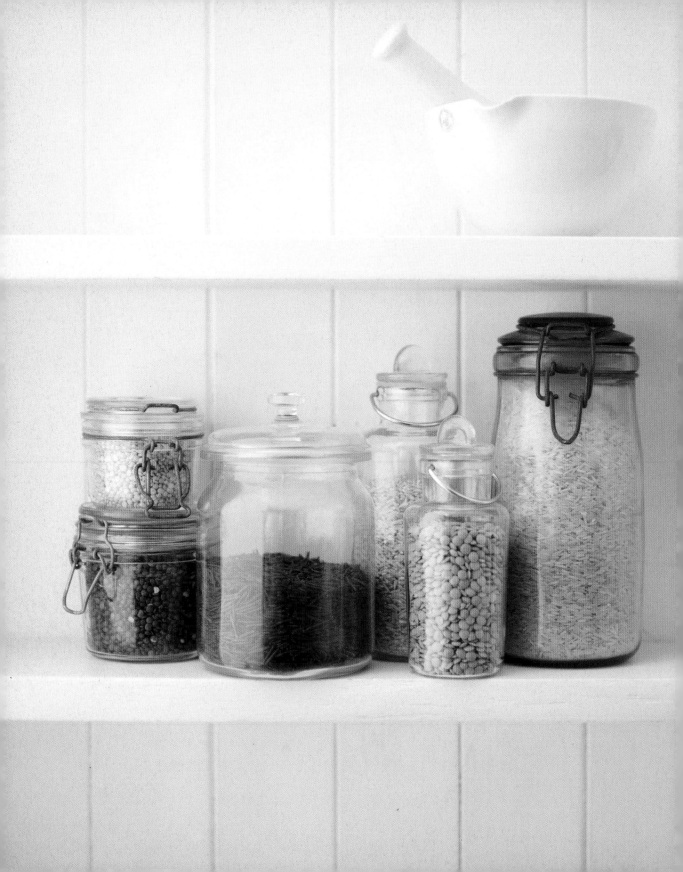

soups

green pea soup

Vivid green, this soup is one of my favourites – for my taste buds and my heart. Peas are packed with folic acid and Vitamin B6, both of which are proven to improve cardiovascular health, and this benefit is not lost when the peas are cooked.

serves 6

1 bouquet garni

3 sprigs of fresh thyme

4 sprigs of fresh parsley

small bunch of fresh mint

2 cloves

1.3kg (3lb) (shelled weight) fresh peas (or use frozen, if not in season)

50g (2oz) spinach

2 Little Gem (Boston) lettuces

1 tbsp olive oil

2 leeks, trimmed and diced

8 celery sticks, finely diced

freshly ground black pepper

low-fat crème fraîche, to serve

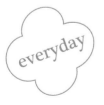

everyday

1 In a large lidded saucepan, bring 2 litres (3½ pints) of unsalted water to the boil. Add the bouquet garni herbs, cloves and peas and simmer for 30 minutes until the peas are very soft.

2 Meanwhile, wash the spinach and remove the stems, and shred the lettuce leaves.

3 Heat the olive oil in a non-stick frying pan set over a medium heat and sauté the leeks and celery for 4 minutes. Then add these to the pea mixture.

4 Finally, add the spinach and lettuce leaves to the soup at the end of the cooking time for the peas and simmer for just 2 more minutes.

5 Don't forget to remove the bouquet garni and herb sprigs before you take the soup off the heat and whiz it up with a hand-held blender.

6 Add a good helping of freshly ground black pepper on top and serve hot with a swirl of low fat crème fraîche.

cauliflower and chickpea soup

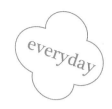
everyday

Cauliflower is a good source of vitamin C and is a member of the cancer-fighting cruciferous family, along with Brussels sprouts and broccoli. This is a gently flavoured soup, even with the curry paste.

serves 4

1 medium onion,
   peeled and diced
2 garlic cloves, peeled
   and crushed
2 tbsp olive oil
1 tbsp cumin seeds
1 litre (1¾ pints/4 cups)
   vegetable stock
1 tsp curry paste
1 small cauliflower,
   cut into small florets
1 x 400g (14oz) tin
   chickpeas, drained
   and rinsed
freshly ground black pepper
fresh coriander (cilantro)
   leaves, to serve
squeeze of fresh lemon
   juice, to serve

1 Gently fry the onion and crushed garlic in olive oil for 4–5 minutes in a large saucepan set over a medium heat, until the onion starts to soften. Add the cumin seeds and fry for another minute.

2 Next, add the vegetable stock and curry paste and bring to the boil. Reduce the heat and add the cauliflower and chickpeas. Simmer over a low heat for 10 minutes or until the cauliflower is tender.

3 Using either a hand-held blender or liquidiser, blend the soup to your desired consistency. Serve with some freshly ground black pepper, a few coriander (cilantro) leaves and a squeeze of fresh lemon if you like.

watercress soup

Watercress is packed with over 15 vitamins and minerals, especially vitamin C, calcium and iron. So enjoy this soup whenever the mood takes you, as it tastes great too!

serves 4

1 tbsp olive oil

1 medium onion, peeled
  and finely chopped

2 garlic cloves, peeled
  and finely chopped

1 tsp curry powder

3 bunches of watercress

900ml (1½ pints/3½ cups)
  vegetable stock

freshly ground black pepper

200g (7oz) low-fat
  fromage frais

1 Heat the olive oil in a medium-sized pan set over a medium heat and sweat the onion until soft. Then add the garlic and cook for 2 minutes. Add the curry powder and cook for another couple of minutes, stirring vigorously.

2 Now, reduce the heat to low, add the watercress and stir for 2 minutes until the watercress wilts. Add the stock, season with black pepper and simmer for 10 minutes.

3 Use a hand-held blender or liquidiser to purée the soup then serve it hot, with plenty of freshly ground black pepper and a swirl of fromage frais in each dish.

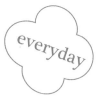
everyday

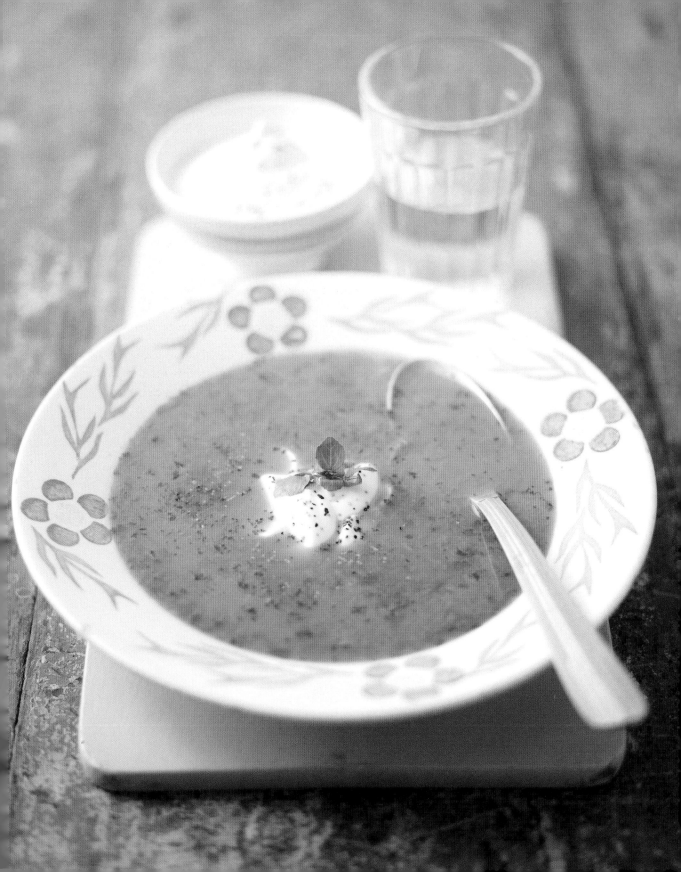

red lentil soup

This is a filling, hearty soup that will keep your hunger pangs at bay – it's filled with fibre and flavour, and is yummy with a spoonful of low-fat natural yogurt and crusty bread. The tomato juice is a great source of vitamins, as are the onions and garlic when cooked with the olive oil.

serves 4–6

1 tbsp olive oil

2 onions, peeled and
    finely chopped

2 celery sticks,
    finely chopped

2 carrots, finely chopped

2 garlic cloves, peeled
    and crushed

2 tsp curry powder

150g (5oz/¾ cup) red lentils

1.5 litres (2½ pints/6⅓ cups)
    vegetable stock

125ml (4½fl oz/½ cup)
    tomato juice

freshly ground black pepper

1 Heat the olive oil in a large pan set over a medium heat, then add the onions, celery and carrots. Cook, stirring, for 5 minutes or until the onions are soft.

2 Add the garlic and curry powder and cook, stirring, for a further 1 minute, then add the lentils, stock and tomato juice.

3 Bring to the boil, then reduce the heat, cover and simmer for 25 minutes or until the vegetables are tender. Take the pan off the heat and purée. You can either whiz up the soup with a hand-held blender or in a liquidiser – or just leave it slightly lumpy if you prefer. Season with freshly ground black pepper and serve hot.

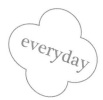

everyday

beetroot soup

Beetroot has long since been used as a medicine to build up patients. It is thought to be a true anti-cancer superfood, filled with anti-carcinogens. The good news for us is that it tastes great too – especially in this really easy to make soup.

everyday

serves 4

400g (14oz) beetroot (beet)

1 tbsp olive oil

1 small onion, peeled and finely chopped

200g (7oz) potatoes, peeled and chopped into small cubes

1 litre (1¾ pints/4 cups) hot vegetable stock

juice of 1 lemon

freshly ground black pepper

2 tbsp low-fat crème fraîche, to serve

2 tbsp chopped chives, to serve

1 Prepare the beetroot (beet) by peeling it and cutting it into 1cm (½in) cubes.

2 Heat the olive oil in a large lidded pan set over a medium heat and add the onion. Cook for 5 minutes until the onion starts to soften. Next, add the beetroot (beet) and potatoes and cook for another 5 minutes.

3 Now add the hot stock, lemon juice and season with freshly ground black pepper and bring to the boil. Reduce the heat and simmer gently, half covered, for about 25 minutes.

4 Allow to cool slightly, then blitz with a hand-held blender or in a liquidiser.

5 Reheat just before serving. Serve with a swirl of the low-fat crème fraîche and a sprinkling of chopped chives.

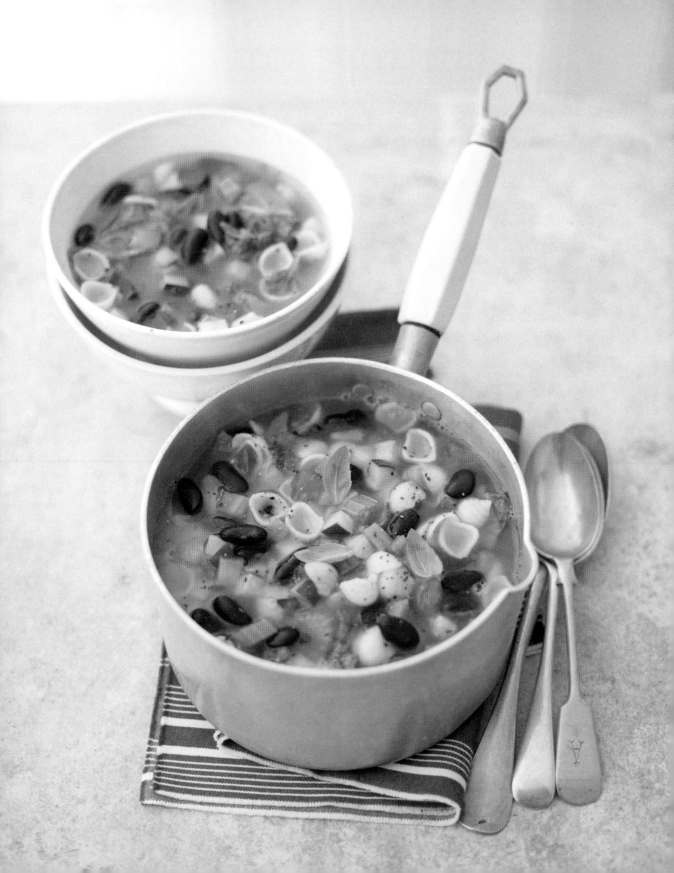

minestrone

This is such an easy recipe, and it provides you with a really filling meal in one bowl.

serves 4

1 tbsp extra-virgin olive oil

1 medium onion, peeled and chopped

2 celery sticks, sliced

1 garlic clove, peeled and crushed

1 carrot, peeled and diced

900ml (1½ pints/3½ cups) chicken stock

2 large tomatoes, deseeded and roughly chopped

1 handful of spinach, chopped

1 x 400g (14oz) tin chickpeas or red kidney beans, drained and rinsed

25g (1oz) uncooked small shell pasta

1 small courgette (zucchini), diced

2 tbsp torn fresh basil leaves

freshly ground black pepper

1 In a large lidded saucepan, heat the olive oil over a medium heat. Add the onion, celery, garlic and carrot and sauté for about 5 minutes until the vegetables have softened.

2 Next, add the stock, tomatoes, spinach, beans and pasta. Bring to the boil over a high heat. Reduce the heat and simmer, covered, for 10 minutes.

3 Finally, add the diced courgettes (zucchini), cover again and cook for 5 minutes more.

4 Remove from the heat, stir in the torn basil leaves and season with freshly ground pepper. Serve immediately.

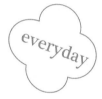

everyday

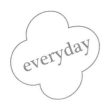

jerusalem artichoke soup

When Jerusalem artichokes are in season, this soup is a must – it is delicious and very quick to make. Serve it with a chunk of wholegrain bread and you've got yourself a quick and nutritious lunch or supper.

serves 4

1 tbsp olive oil

500g (1lb 2oz) Jerusalem artichokes, thinly sliced

1 medium onion, peeled and finely chopped

1 medium potato, peeled and finely diced

1 garlic clove, peeled and chopped

900ml (1½ pints/3½ cups) vegetable stock

1 small bunch of watercress, trimmed

2 tbsp finely chopped fresh parsley

1 Heat the olive oil in a large saucepan set over a medium heat, then add the artichokes, onion, potato and garlic and sauté for 3–4 minutes, until the onion is just transparent but not browned.

2 Next, add the stock and simmer for 10–15 minutes until the artichoke pieces are soft and tender.

3 Add the watercress and cook for another 4 minutes. Take off the heat and use a hand-held blender or liquidiser to purée the soup.

4 Reheat and sprinkle on the chopped parsley just before serving.

roasted tomato soup

Simple, classic and very tasty, this dish also happens to be great for your heart.

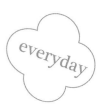
everyday

serves 4

1kg (2lb 2oz) tomatoes

3 garlic cloves, peeled and
  crushed

2 tbsp dried mixed herbs

freshly ground black pepper

2 tbsp olive oil

600ml (1 pint/2½ cups) hot
  vegetable stock

2 tsp balsamic vinegar

1 Preheat the oven to 180°C/350°F/Gas mark 4.

2 Wash the tomatoes and cut each one in half. Place them
  on a roasting tray and sprinkle over the crushed garlic,
  dried herbs, freshly ground black pepper and the olive
  oil. Roast for about 1 hour or until the tomatoes are
  starting to brown at the edges.

3 Remove from the oven and, once the tomatoes
  have cooled slightly, transfer to a large saucepan.
  Add the stock and balsamic vinegar. Whiz up with
  a hand-held blender, then heat through once more
  before serving.

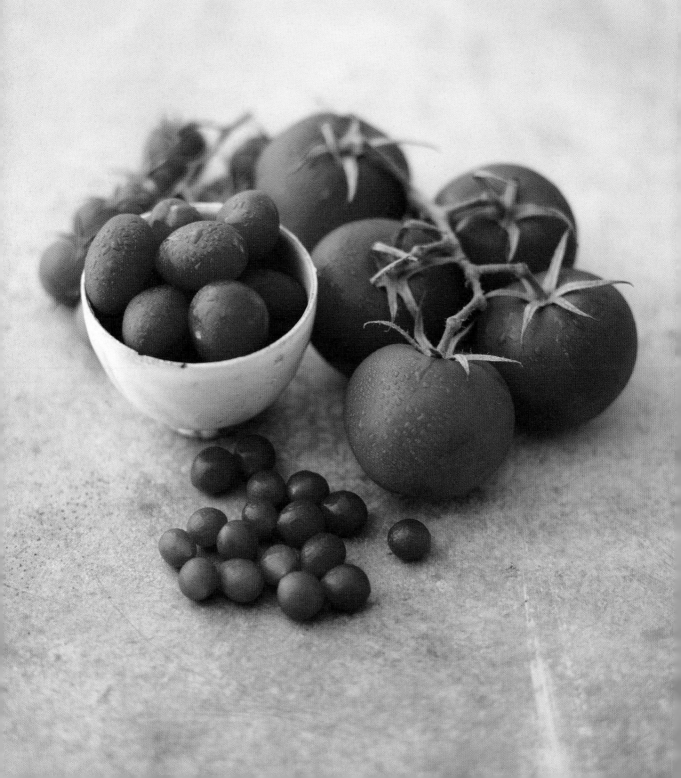

salads

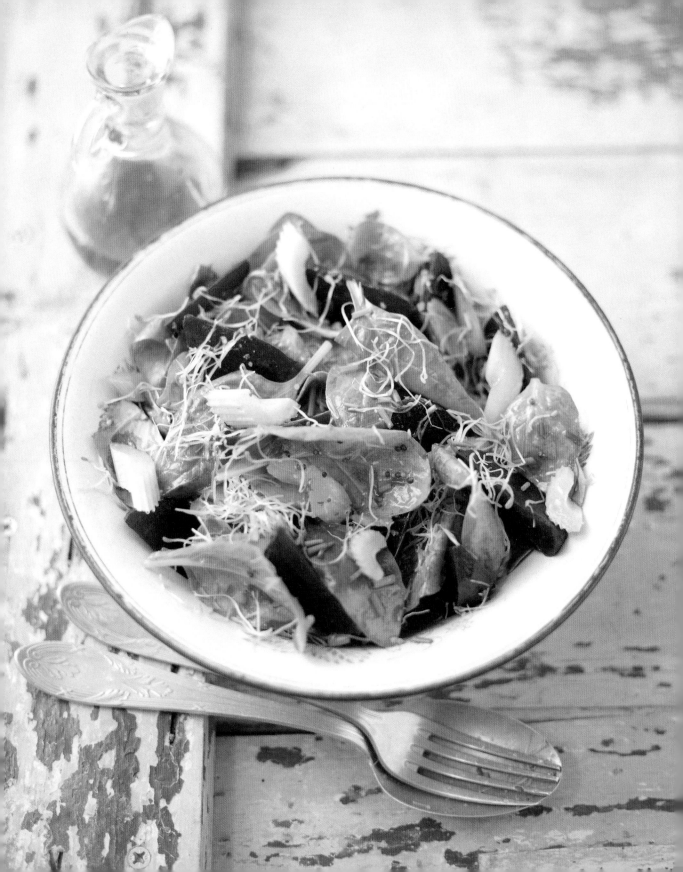

beetroot and spinach superfood salad

Beetroot is jam-packed full of great vitamins and minerals, including iron, calcium, vitamin B6 and potassium. It helps you fight off infection and is also thought to protect against some cancers. So this dish provides a powerful health boost that tastes great. Put the salad together just before serving so that the beetroot doesn't stain all the other ingredients.

serves
2 as a main course,
4 as a side dish

for the salad

100g (3½oz) baby spinach leaves

75g (3oz/2¼ cups) alfalfa sprouts

2 celery sticks, sliced

4 cooked beetroot, each cut into 8 wedges

for the dressing

4 tbsp olive oil

1½ tbsp garlic wine vinegar

1 tsp wholegrain mustard

1 garlic clove, peeled and crushed

2 tsp clear honey

1 tbsp snipped chives

1 tbsp chopped fresh parsley

1 To make the dressing, mix the all the dressing ingredients together in a bowl. Set aside.

2 Put the spinach, alfalfa sprouts and celery in another bowl and mix together. Now add in the beetroot and mix well. Pour the dressing over the salad, toss well and serve immediately.

Tip:

I like to buy fresh beetroot when available from my local farmers' market. I chop the stalks off the top, then boil the beetroot for about an hour. Alternatively, you can buy ready-cooked beetroot from your supermarket, vacuum packed.

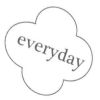

everyday

bacon, egg and asparagus salad

Quick to put together, this salad makes an impressive little starter or light brunch.

serves 2

2 rashers of bacon

250g (9oz) asparagus, woody ends snapped off

150g (5oz) broad (fava) beans

2 eggs

200g (7oz) watercress

3 tbsp low-fat shop-bought French dressing

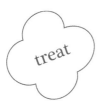

treat

1 Preheat the grill (broiler) to medium.

2 Cut all visible fat off the bacon, then grill (broil) the bacon until it's nice and crispy. Set aside.

3 Cook the asparagus in a large pan of boiling water or 2 minutes. Add the broad (fava) beans and simmer for a further 3 minutes until both the beans and asparagus are tender. Drain and set aside.

4 To poach the eggs, bring a large pan of water to the boil. Crack the first egg into a teacup then gently slip the egg into the water. Do the same with the remaining egg then simmer very gently for 1 minute. Turn off the heat, cover and leave to stand for 5 minutes until the eggs are just set.

5 While the eggs are cooking, toss the watercress and cooled beans and asparagus lightly in 2 tablespoons of the salad dressing and divide between 2 bowls.

6 Lift the eggs from the water using a slotted spoon, drain well, then place one on top of each salad.

7 Break the bacon into pieces and scatter over the top. Drizzle the remaining tablespoon of dressing over and serve straight away with warmed, crusty wholegrain bread.

beansprout, carrot and courgette salad

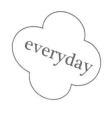
everyday

Light, colourful and nutritious. Serve this salad as a main course or a side dish to get the full nutritional benefit.

serves 6

for the salad

275g (10oz/2½ cups) grated carrot

225g (8oz/1⅛ cups) grated courgette (zucchini)

175g (6oz/¾ cup) beansprouts

1 red (bell) pepper, deseeded and finely sliced

85g (3oz/½ cup) frozen sweetcorn (corn), thawed

3 tbsp pumpkin seeds

3 tbsp sunflower seeds

for the dressing

2 tbsp olive oil

juice of 1 lemon

1 tbsp balsamic vinegar

1 tsp wholegrain mustard

1 Combine all the salad ingredients in a large serving bowl.

2 To make the dressing, simply whisk together all the dressing ingredients in a bowl.

3 Pour the dressing over the salad and serve.

Tip:

It's important that you serve a salad as soon as you've prepared it. The longer it has been 'cut', the more nutrients are lost. And anyway … it tastes so good – why wait?

smoked mackerel citrus salad

Besides being deliciously tasty, mackerel is also high in omega-3, which is essential for good health. This simple salad provides you with a perfectly balanced meal that can be enjoyed any time, anywhere.

serves
2 as a main course
or 4 as a side dish

for the salad

200g (7oz) green beans

200g (7oz) smoked
mackerel fillets

125g (4½oz) mixed
watercress, spinach and
rocket

4 spring onions (scallions),
sliced

½ cucumber, diced

2 tbsp sunflower seeds

1 avocado, sliced

for the dressing

1 tbsp olive oil

1 tbsp chopped fresh
coriander (cilantro)

freshly ground black pepper

zest and juice of 1 orange

juice of ½ lemon

1 Preheat the grill (broiler) to medium.

2 Blanch the green beans in boiling water for 3 minutes until they are just tender, then drain well and refresh under cold water. Set aside.

3 Grill (broil) the mackerel for 2 minutes just to warm them through. Then peel back the skin, discard it, and cut the flesh into 2cm (¾in) pieces.

4 Place the salad leaves in a bowl with the spring onions (scallions), cucumber, sunflower seeds and avocado, then add the fish.

5 In a separate bowl, mix the olive oil with the coriander (cilantro), freshly ground black pepper, orange zest and juice and lemon juice.

6 Pour the dressing over the salad, toss together well and serve immediately.

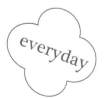

everyday

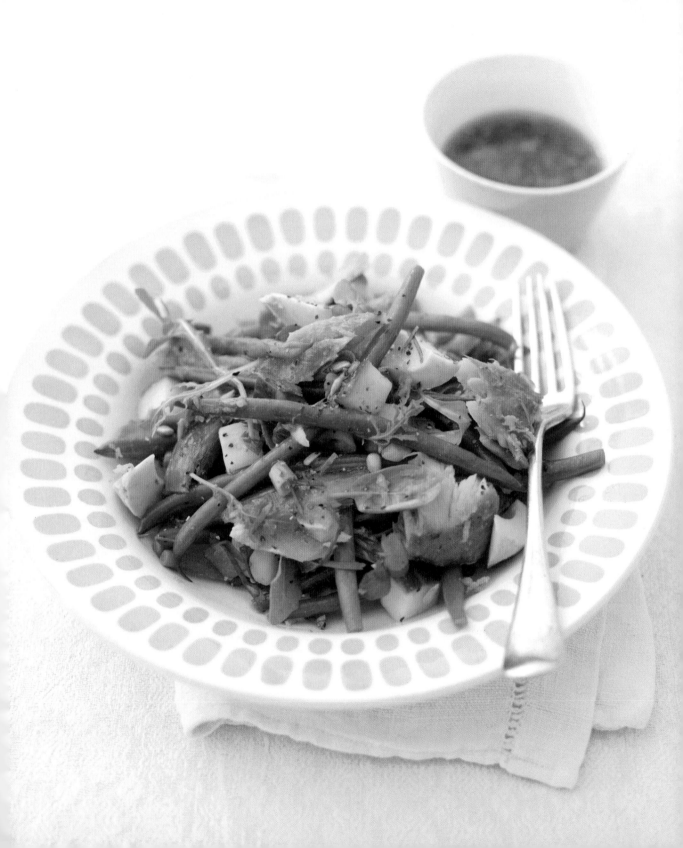

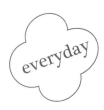

warm mushroom salad

Salads get a bad press and are often accused of being boring Well, this salad is far from boring – in fact, it is a filling, warming meal, packed with goodness. The raw spinach and watercress are iron-rich and are proven to provide a great barrier for some cancers. The cloves, garlic and paprika provide good flavour, and the mushrooms make this a wonderful, textured and satisfying meal.

serves 4

300g (11oz) packet of
  spinach and watercress
250g (9oz) large brown
  chestnut (cremini)
  mushrooms
250g (9oz) mixed wild
  mushrooms
1 tbsp olive oil
2 tbsp pine nuts
3 cloves
2 garlic cloves, peeled and
  crushed
freshly ground black pepper
150ml (5fl oz/⅔ cup)
  white wine
4 tbsp balsamic vinegar
sprinkling of paprika,
  to serve
handful of chopped fresh
  flat-leaf parsley, to serve

1 Wash and dry the spinach and watercress leaves and put them in a bowl.

2 Brush clean the mushrooms, skimming the top skin off, if necessary. Cut each mushroom into quarters if large, but leave them whole if small.

3 In a large frying pan set over a high heat, fry all the mushrooms in the olive oil with the pine nuts, cloves, garlic and freshly ground black pepper for 2–3 minutes.

4 Add the white wine and balsamic vinegar and cook down for another 3 minutes. Then pour over the washed spinach and watercress, sprinkle with paprika and chopped parsley and serve straight away while still warm.

american broccoli salad

Broccoli is a true superfood. It is an excellent source of fibre, folate, vitamins A, C, B2, B6, potassium, iron and calcium – phew! Therefore I have happily marked this as an everyday dish even though there is some salt in the very lean bacon. Although broccoli is one of the best foods you can eat, it's important to make it tasty and enticing, so that you can eat lots of it. I've substituted low-fat crème fraîche for the usual high-fat mayonnaise and, along with the tart flavour of the apple cider vinegar, this lovely adapted American recipe works really well.

serves 4

8 slices of very lean back (Canadian) bacon

1 large head of broccoli, cut into florets

75g (3oz) red seedless grapes, halved

2 red onions, peeled and finely sliced

160g (5½oz/⅔ cup) low-fat crème fraîche

2 tbsp apple cider vinegar

25g (1oz/¼ cup) flaked (slivered) almonds, toasted

75g (3oz/½ cup) raisins

1 Preheat the grill (broiler) to medium.

2 Cut all visible fat off the bacon and grill (broil) the bacon until it's nice and crispy. Once cooked, cut up into bite-size pieces and set aside.

3 In a large bowl, combine the broccoli, grapes and onions.

4 Whisk the low-fat crème fraîche and apple cider vinegar together. Toss this with broccoli mixture and chill.

5 Just before serving, toss the bacon, almonds and raisins through the salad and serve.

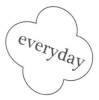
everyday

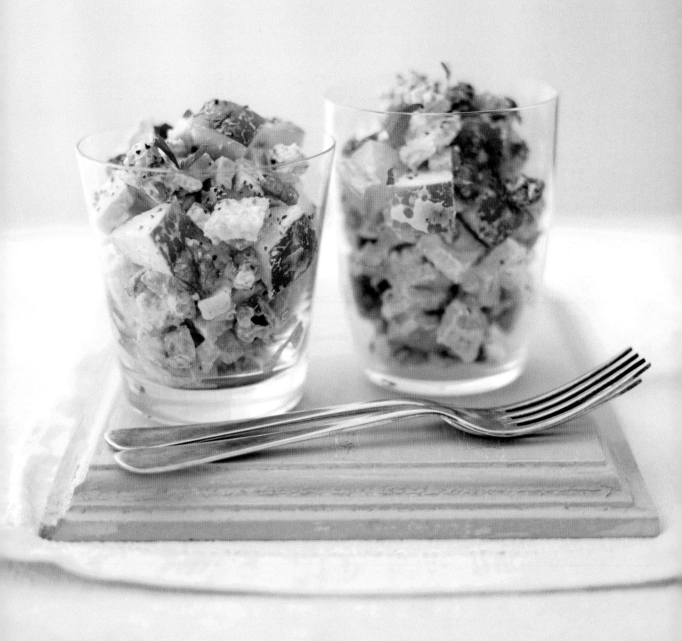

turkey waldorf salad

This recipe is great for using up any leftover cold turkey but feel free to swap the turkey for cold, cooked chicken or even tinned tuna fish. You'll notice the usual creamy mayonnaise dressing has been swapped for a low-fat choice, which works just as well.

serves 4

for the salad

4 celery sticks, chopped

2 eating apples, unpeeled, cored and chopped

small handful of raisins

60g (2oz/½ cup) walnuts, chopped (try to buy organic – they taste amazing!)

2 handfuls of leftover cold turkey, chopped

1 tbsp chopped fresh parsley

for the dressing

juice of ½ lemon

150g (5oz/⅔ cup) natural low-fat thick yogurt

1 tbsp olive oil

freshly ground black pepper

1 Place the celery, apples, raisins, walnuts and meat (or fish, if using an alternative to turkey) in a large salad serving bowl.

2 In a separate bowl, mix together the lemon juice, yogurt, olive oil and season with freshly ground black pepper, then mix the dressing into the salad and toss through. Sprinkle with chopped parsley and serve.

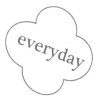

everyday

crunchy bean salad

This is a feisty salad! The fennel gives it a lovely aniseed flavour, and the radishes give it a lively kick. It's actually my favourite salad of all – I hope you love it, too.

serves 4

4–5 Chinese leaves, to line the serving bowl (or iceberg lettuce will do)

1 fennel bulb, trimmed, sliced

5–6 radishes, sliced

1 small green apple, sliced

½ courgette (zucchini), thinly sliced

2 shallots, peeled and finely diced

200g (7oz) edamame beans, blanched

250g (9oz) French (green) beans, blanched

handful of chopped fresh parsley

handful of chopped fresh lemon thyme leaves

zest and juice of 1 large lemon

glug of olive oil

glug of balsamic vinegar

freshly ground black pepper

1 Use the Chinese leaves to line a serving bowl. Set aside.

2 In a large bowl, mix together the fennel, radishes, apple, courgette (zucchini), shallots, both types of beans and herbs. Now mix it all up with the lemon zest and juice, olive oil, balsamic vinegar and a good sprinkling of freshly ground black pepper.

3 Transfer the salad to the bowl lined with Chinese leaves to serve.

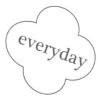

everyday

winter salad

Quick, deliciously tasty and healthy – who ever said that salads were boring?

serves 4

for the salad

½ crisp white cabbage,
  sliced

1 large fennel bulb, sliced

2 celery sticks, sliced

3 white radishes, sliced

1 apple, peeled, cored and
  chopped

1 handful of chopped fresh
  parsley

for the dressing

2 tbsp olive oil

1 tbsp lemon juice

freshly ground black pepper

1 Wash and prepare all the salad ingredients except the parsley and put into a large shallow serving dish.

2 In a separate bowl, mix the olive oil, lemon juice and freshly ground black pepper and pour over the salad. Now sprinkle with the chopped parsley and serve.

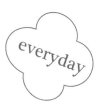

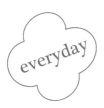

white haricot bean and tomato salad

I absolutely adore this salad. Try to serve it while the potatoes are still just warm. Haricot beans are a brilliant source of protein, fibre and iron and are inexpensive, too!

serves 6

400g (14oz) waxy new
   potatoes

400g (14oz) ripe tomatoes

12 black olives, pitted and
   halved

2 x 410g (14oz) tins white
   haricot beans, drained

4 spring onions (scallions),
   finely sliced

1 bunch of fresh flat-leaf
   parsley, roughly chopped

1 red chilli, deseeded,
   finely diced

4 tbsp extra virgin olive oil

zest and juice of 1 lemon

freshly ground black pepper

1 Boil the potatoes in their skins in a large pan set over a high heat for 20 minutes. Drain and, as soon as they are cool enough to handle, cut them into wedges.

2 Dip the tomatoes in a pan of boiling water for 20 seconds, peel them, then cut them into wedges. Remove the seeds.

3 Mix the potatoes, tomatoes, black olives and beans together in a bowl. In another bowl, combine the spring onions (scallions), parsley and chilli with the olive oil, lemon zest and juice and freshly ground black pepper to taste, and pour this dressing over the tomatoes, beans and potatoes. Mix well and serve immediately, while the potatoes are still warm.

Tip:

I'll let you into a little secret: I don't always do the whole dipping and skinning thing with the tomatoes. If I do have time I do it, I love the results – the tomatoes take on the flavours of the other ingredients and really soften up. But if you are in a hurry, don't let that step put you off – just slice the tomatoes up as usual.

warm lentil salad

Lentils are rich in protein, minerals and fibre and are a good source of B vitamins – plus they are recommended by cardiologists the world over. So this delicious, warming salad ticks all the right boxes. I like to use red lentils for this recipe, but you can use your favourite.

serves 4

1 tbsp olive oil

1 onion, peeled and finely chopped

1 garlic clove, peeled and chopped

1 carrot, peeled, finely chopped

1 celery stick, finely chopped

2 red (bell) peppers, deseeded and roughly chopped

200g (7oz) flat mushrooms, sliced

225g (8oz/1⅛ cups) lentils, rinsed and drained

600ml (1 pint/2½ cups) hot vegetable stock

100g (3½oz) spinach

freshly ground black pepper

2 tbsp balsamic vinegar

1 Heat the olive oil in a large non-stick lidded pan and add the onion, garlic, carrot and celery pieces. Cook for about 5 minutes until the vegetables begin to soften.

2 Next, add the chopped (bell) peppers and sliced mushrooms, cover and cook for a further 5 minutes.

3 Now stir in the rinsed lentils and hot stock. Bring to the boil, then reduce the heat a little and simmer, covered, for 25–30 minutes.

4 A couple of minutes before the end of the cooking time, add the spinach and freshly ground black pepper to taste and cook until the spinach has wilted.

5 Finally, stir in the balsamic vinegar, then serve.

Tip:
If you want to make this a larger meal, serve it with a poached egg sitting on top of the salad – a delicious addition!

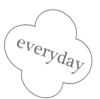

everyday

asparagus & artichoke salad with wild rice & basil dressing

During the asparagus season, make the most of their full flavour and enjoy.

serves 4

for the salad

125g (4½oz/⅝ cup) wild rice

4 globe artichokes

juice of 1 lemon

1 large bunch of asparagus

1 tbsp olive oil

1 tbsp lime juice

1 garlic clove, peeled and crushed

freshly ground black pepper

¼ red (bell) pepper, finely diced, to garnish

for the basil dressing

1 tbsp wholegrain mustard

1 handful of basil leaves, shredded

1 tbsp olive oil

1 garlic clove, peeled and crushed

juice of 1 lemon

freshly ground black pepper

1 Cook the wild rice for about 45 minutes or until soft and the grains are bursting. Drain well and set aside.

2 While the rice is cooking, trim the artichokes and add them to a large saucepan of boiling water with the lemon juice. Boil over a high heat for 25 minutes or until tender. Refresh in cold water and leave to drain upside down. Then remove the outer leaves and any woody stalks and scrape out the hairy choke. Cut the artichokes into wedges.

3 Next, blanch the asparagus in boiling water for 1–2 minutes, depending on its thickness, until just tender. Refresh in cold water and drain well.

4 Place the artichoke wedges and asparagus in a large bowl and add the olive oil, lime juice, garlic and freshly ground black pepper and mix together well. Set aside to marinate for about 10 minutes.

5 Now, in a small bowl, mix together all the ingredients for the basil dressing and set aside.

6 Preheat the grill (broiler) to medium. Put the marinated artichoke and asparagus on a flat grill (broiler) pan and grill (broil) until lightly charred.

7 Finally, toss the grilled (broiled) vegetables with the rice and the basil dressing and garnish with the raw diced red (bell) pepper.

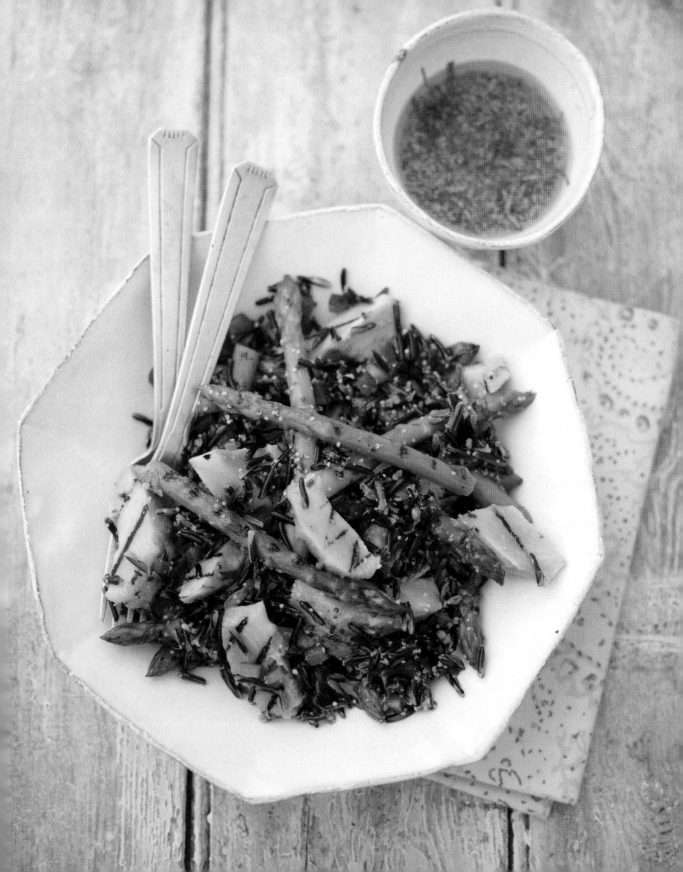

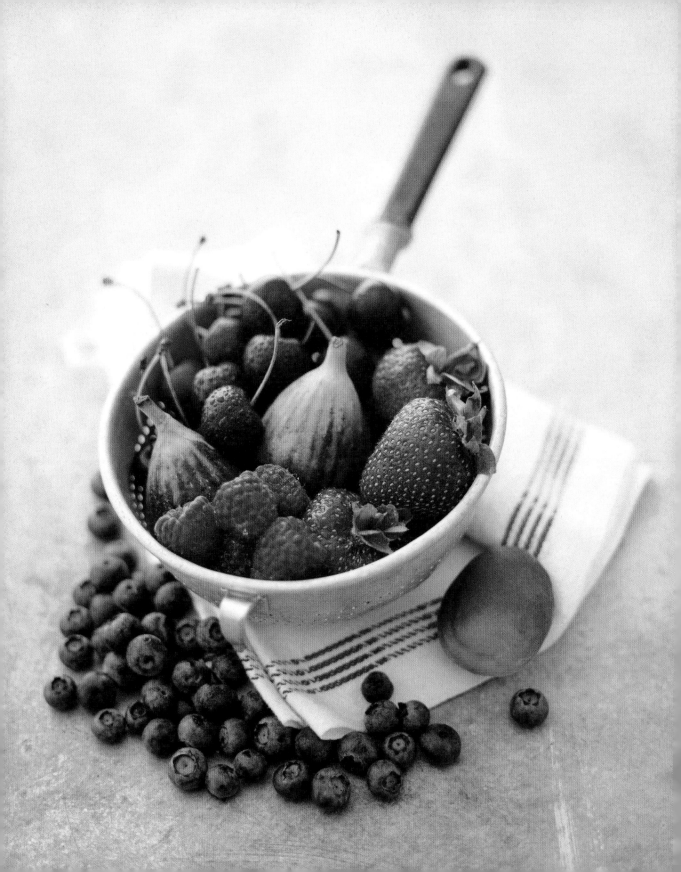

sides
&
starters

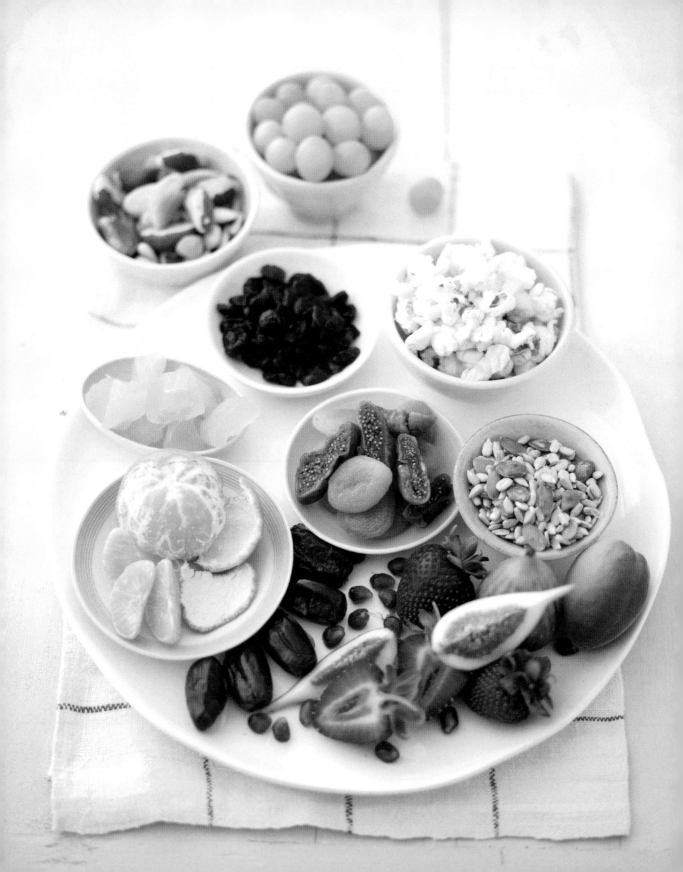

fruit and nut mezze

Encouraging children to try new foods can be quite a challenge. Try waiting until they are really hungry, then put a healthy 'mezze' (a collection of small dishes or starters) on the table and let them experiment. You can keep it interesting by changing the ingredients each time you serve it. Be as imaginative as you like about what you use – there are many fresh and dried fruits, and nuts and seeds etc, to choose from. The list of ideas for ingredients below will help you get started. Serve up the mezze in small bowls that will catch the attention of your children.

everyday

serves 4

fresh fruit
sliced banana
pineapple, cubed
strawberries
apricots
apples, sliced
figs
tangerine segments
grapes
pomegranate seeds

nuts and seeds
blanched whole
  almonds
Brazil nuts
macadamia nuts
sunflower seeds
pumpkin seeds

dried fruit
dried cranberries
mixed soft dried
  fruit
soft dried dates
soft figs

other
unsalted popcorn
olives

Tip:
Don't be afraid to throw little bowls of chocolate buttons and sweeties into the mix on occasions. I believe that guilt shouldn't be attached to treats – rather, they should be savoured, as long as the nutritious food comes first.

heart-healthy slow-cooked onions

Cardiologists find onions fascinating! After many studies it has been confirmed that both onions and garlic can protect the circulatory system and can help with the symptoms of anaemia, arthritis and rheumatism … They taste good, too! This wonderful side dish needs a little marinating time in advance.

serves 4

5 tbsp olive oil

pinch of saffron

½ tsp ground ginger

1 tsp freshly ground black pepper

1 tsp ground cinnamon

1 tbsp granulated sugar

700g (1½lb) Spanish or red onions

4 garlic cloves, peeled

1 In a bowl, mix up the olive oil, saffron, ground ginger, black pepper, cinnamon and sugar. Set aside.

2 Peel and slice the onions and place in a lidded casserole dish or ovenproof dish with the garlic.

3 Pour the oil-and-spice mixture over the onions, ensuring all the onions are well covered in the oil, and leave to marinate, preferably for about 2 hours.

4 Preheat the oven to 170°C/325°F/Gas mark 3.

5 After marinating, cover with foil and the lid of the casserole dish and bake for 45 minutes or until the onions are very soft, then increase the oven temperature to 200°C/400°F/Gas mark 6. Remove the lid and foil and cook for a further 5–10 minutes or until the onions are lightly glazed. Serve immediately.

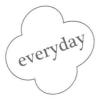
everyday

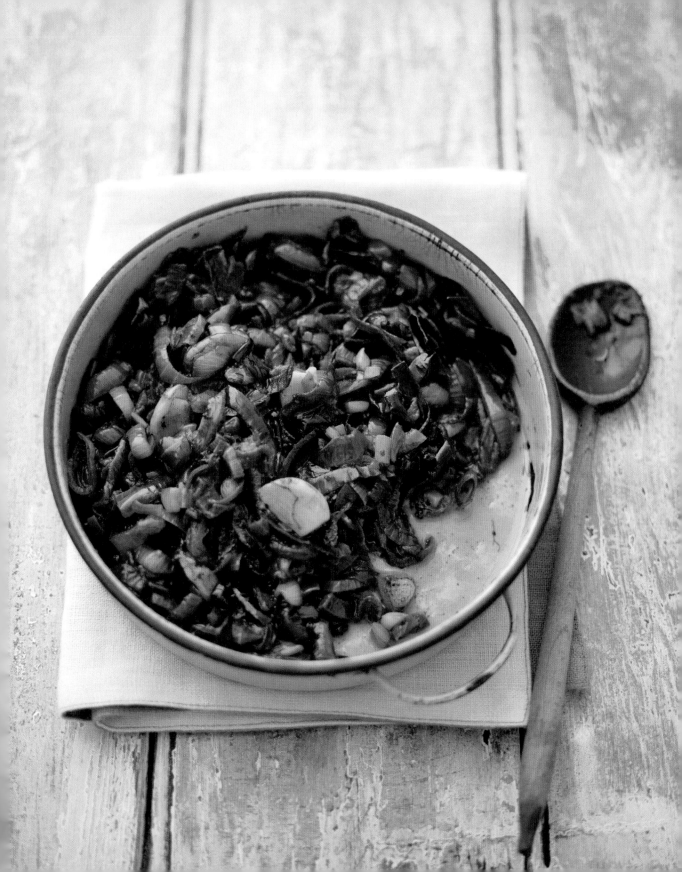

thai fragrant rice

Learning how to make delicious rice will make feeding you and your family easier. Rice is fat free, and is a good carbohydrate food that will help to steady blood sugar levels, making it less likely that you'll have hunger pangs or sweet cravings between meals. It goes without saying that brown rice would usually be the preferred healthy choice, but there isn't always time to wait for it to cook. This is a quicker and much healthier option than chips! Basmati rice is cooked with lemongrass, fresh ginger and spices to make a wonderfully aromatic fluffy rice. My children are always nicely filled up when I give them this rice with one of my vegetable stir-fries.

serves 4

2 cloves

1 stick of lemongrass, bruised and halved

2.5cm (1in) fresh ginger, peeled and sliced

2 tsp ground nutmeg

1 cinnamon stick

1 bay leaf

2 small, thin strips of lime zest

350g (12oz/1¾ cups) basmati rice

freshly ground black pepper

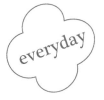

1 Put the cloves, lemongrass, ginger, nutmeg, cinnamon stick, bay leaf and lime zest in a large lidded heavy-based saucepan with 600ml (1 pint/2½ cups) water and bring to the boil over a high heat.

2 Reduce the heat to a medium–low and add the rice. Stir well, then cover and simmer for 10–15 minutes or until all the liquid has been absorbed and the rice is nice and tender, but still has a bite to it.

3 Remove the saucepan from the heat, add freshly ground black pepper to taste, then fluff up the rice with a fork. Remove any of the large pieces of the spices and the lemongrass before serving.

avocado salsa

This tasty, nutritious side dish works well with a barbecue, and can be served with some toasted wholemeal pitta bread as a snack or starter.

serves 4

1 avocado

1 green chilli, deseeded
   and diced

1 red (bell) pepper,
   deseeded and diced

2 tbsp chopped fresh
   coriander (cilantro)

freshly ground black pepper

juice of 1 lime

1 Peel the avocado and cut into small cubes. Place in a large bowl.

2 Add the diced green chilli, red (bell) pepper and coriander (cilantro).

3 Season with black pepper, add the lime juice, toss well and serve.

everyday

parsnip chippies

This is a delicious, healthy alternative to crisps (potato chips) – great for the kids when they get in from school, or as a snack while on the go.

serves 4

for the chippies

4 tsp coriander seeds

4 tsp cumin seeds

4 parsnips, peeled, cut into 0.5cm (¼in) wide matchsticks

1 tbsp olive oil

for the dip

125g (4½oz/½ cup) low-fat thick Greek yogurt

juice of 1 lemon

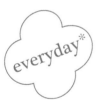
everyday*

1 Preheat the oven to 200°C/400°F/Gas mark 6.

2 Place the coriander and cumin seeds into a dry frying pan and toast them over a high heat for about 2 minutes, stirring continuously, until you start to smell their aroma and they begin to change colour. Then transfer to a pestle and mortar and crush down gently.

3 Now place the parsnip matchsticks into a large bowl and drizzle over the olive oil, mixing well. Shake the crushed toasted spices over them and mix really well, so that the parsnips are all well dusted.

4 Pour the parsnips on to a non-stick baking tray and cook for 15–20 minutes until slightly browned at the edges.

5 Meanwhile, pour the yogurt into a small bowl and stir in the lemon juice. Set aside. Serve the yogurt alongside the parsnip chippies as a dip. The avocado salsa (see p67) also goes well with the parsnip chippies.

* This is an everyday dish only without the dip – with the yogurt, it becomes a treat.

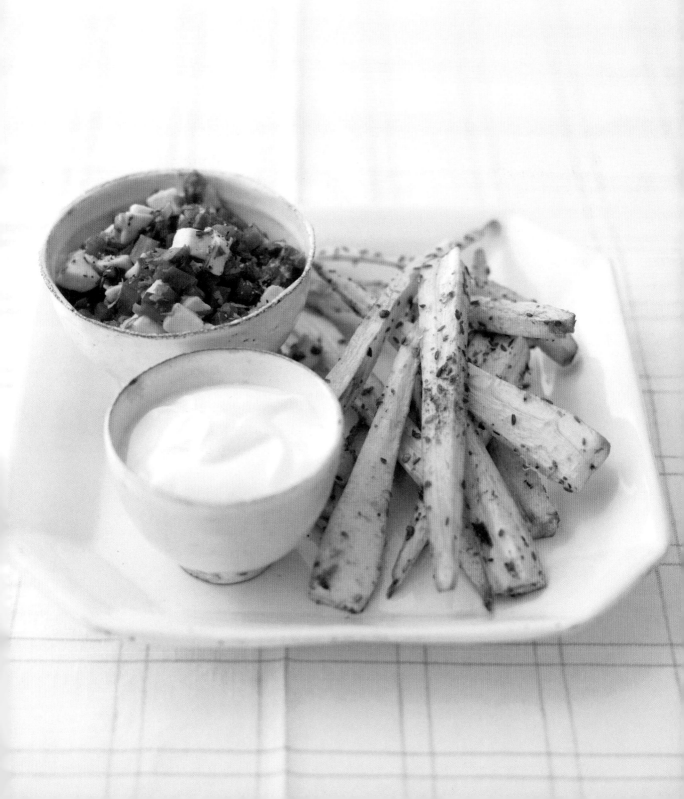

ratatouille

Serve this as a side dish to accompany, chicken, fish or red meat. Packed with antioxidants and vitamins, this is a must-have dish for nutrient boosting!

serves 4

2 courgettes (zucchini)

2 small aubergines (eggplants)

2 tbsp olive oil

1 large onion, peeled and sliced

1 garlic clove, peeled and crushed

1 green (bell) pepper, deseeded and sliced

1 red (bell) pepper, deseeded and sliced

6 tomatoes, quartered

2 glugs Worcestershire sauce

2 tsp sugar

pinch of ground coriander

freshly ground black pepper

1 tbsp chopped fresh basil, to serve

1 Wash the courgettes (zucchini) and aubergines (eggplants) and cut into bite-size pieces.

2 Heat 1 tablespoon of the olive oil in a large lidded heavy-based saucepan set over a medium heat and cook the onion and garlic for about 5 minutes until soft.

3 Next, add the aubergine (eggplant) and fry until soft but not brown.

4 Add the other tablespoon of olive oil and add the (bell) peppers and courgettes (zucchini), cover and cook over a low heat for 25 minutes.

5 Add the tomatoes, Worcestershire sauce, sugar, coriander and black pepper to taste, and then cook, covered, for another 20 minutes.

6 Sprinkle with some chopped basil and serve hot.

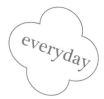

vegetable sauce

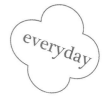

everyday

This is a lovely, delicate sauce that will work well poured over some cooked fish or chicken just before you serve up. It will keep for a week in the refrigerator, and will heat up beautifully each time you want to use some.

serves 4

1 tbsp olive oil

¼ onion, peeled and diced

½ leek, diced

½ celery stick, trimmed and diced

30g (1oz) carrots, peeled and diced

30g (1oz) white cabbage, shredded

½ tsp crushed garlic

½ tsp crushed black peppercorns

150ml (5fl oz/⅔ cups) dry white wine

2 tbsp low-fat crème fraîche

1 Heat the olive oil in a medium-sized lidded saucepan set over a medium heat. Add the vegetables and garlic, cover with the lid and sweat gently for about 10 minutes or until soft.

2 Add the peppercorns and the wine, bring to the boil, then simmer, uncovered, until reduced by about half. Add 300ml (10fl oz/1¼ cups) water and bring to the boil, then reduce the heat to simmer gently for 20–25 minutes.

3 Take off the heat and pass the vegetables through a fine sieve. Skim off any fat that rises to the top, then stir in the crème fraîche and serve.

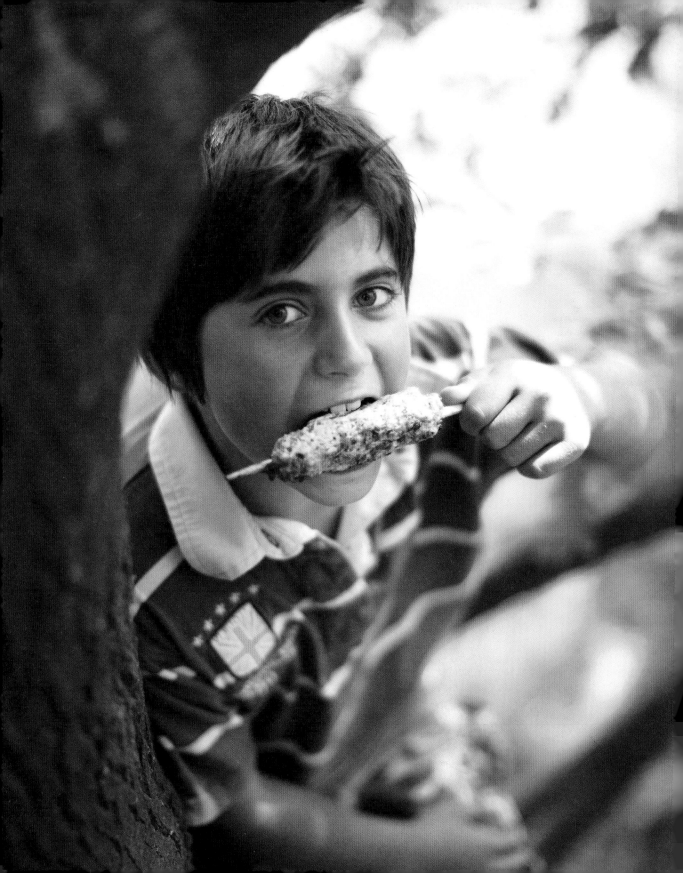

chicken
&
turkey

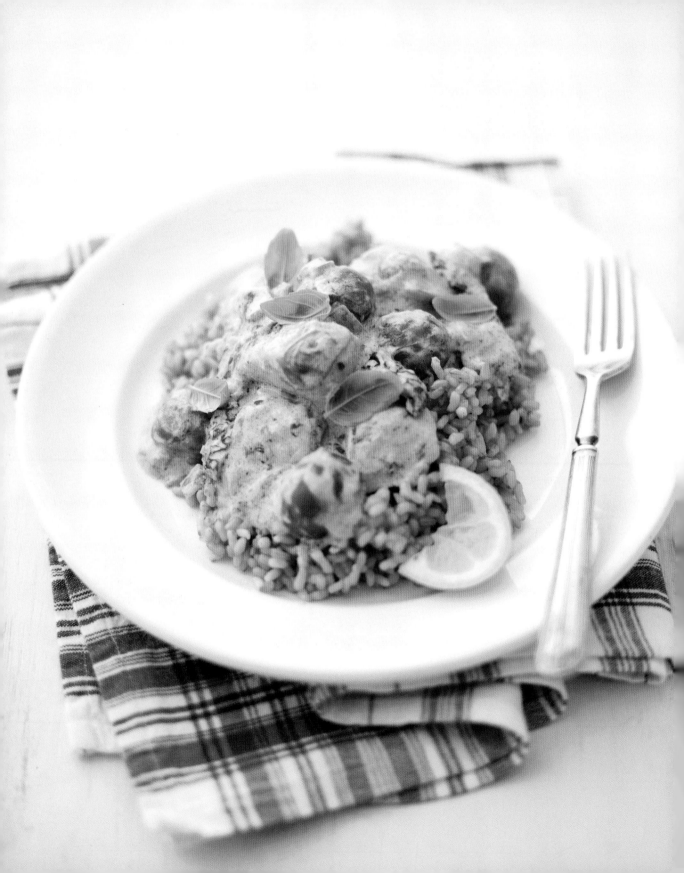

speedy cherry tomatoes and chicken

This dish contains two kinds of tomatoes for added taste and health benefit. Tomatoes are rich in antioxidants, particularly betacarotene and lycopene, and vitamins C and E. It's important to note that this dish contains sun-dried tomatoes. These days, some processed tomatoes can contain more lycopene than fresh ones, so don't be put off by tinned and sun-dried tomatoes or tomato sauces – they will still give you all the healthy benefits that you deserve!

serves 4

2 tbsp olive oil

juice of ½ lemon

175g (6oz/¾ cup) short-grain brown rice (cooked as per packet instructions)

4 skinless chicken breast fillets, cut into 2.5cm (1in) cubes

2 garlic cloves, peeled and crushed

1 onion, peeled and finely chopped

1 tbsp green pesto

12 sun-dried tomatoes, halved

20 cherry tomatoes

400ml (14fl oz/1¾ cups) low-fat crème fraîche

freshly ground black pepper

3–4 fresh basil leaves, torn, to serve

lemon wedges, to serve

1 To cook the rice, put 600ml (1 pint) water in a large lidded saucepan, bring to the boil and add 1 tablespoon of the olive oil and the lemon juice. Add the rice and cook as per the packet instructions.

2 Meanwhile, in a large, non-stick frying pan, add the other tablespoon of olive oil and the chicken. Over a medium heat, brown the chicken on all sides, cooking for about 4 minutes.

3 Next add the garlic, onion, pesto and both types of tomatoes and, stirring continuously, cook for about 5 minutes until the tomatoes start to soften.

4 Ensure the chicken is cooked through (check by cutting one of the chunks in half), then add the crème fraîche and stir through. Season with freshly ground black pepper.

5 Serve immediately with the cooked rice and some torn basil leaves scattered over.

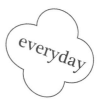
everyday

chicken 'n' rice

This lovely, colourful chicken dish is conveniently cooked in one pot, and you can easily increase the ingredients to feed a houseful!

serves 4

4 tbsp olive oil

4 skinless, boneless chicken breasts

1 large onion, peeled and finely sliced

1 green (bell) pepper, deseeded and chopped

1 red (bell) pepper, deseeded and chopped

1 yellow (bell) pepper, deseeded and chopped

2 garlic cloves, peeled and finely chopped

1 tsp paprika

2 bay leaves

1 x 400g (14oz) tin chopped tomatoes

1 tsp fresh thyme leaves

1 tsp dried oregano

175g (6oz/¾ cup) long-grain rice

750ml (1¼ pints/3 cups) chicken or vegetable stock

4 tbsp tomato purée (paste)

juice of 1 lemon

freshly ground black pepper

100g (3½oz/¾ cup) frozen peas

1 Preheat the oven to 180°C/350°F/Gas mark 4.

2 In a large lidded flameproof casserole dish set over a high heat, add 2 tablespoons of the olive oil and fry the chicken breasts, turning frequently, for 4–5 minutes or until evenly browned. Remove from the casserole dish and set aside.

3 Add the remaining oil to the casserole dish, reduce the heat to medium heat and fry the onion until softened. Add the chopped (bell) peppers and garlic and fry for 5 minutes or until the (bell) peppers start to soften. Add the paprika, bay leaves, tomatoes, thyme and oregano and stir in the rice. Fry for 1–2 minutes, stirring constantly.

4 Next, add the chicken or vegetable stock, tomato purée, lemon juice and season to taste with freshly ground black pepper.

5 Return the chicken breasts to the casserole, pushing them down into the rice, cover and cook in the oven for 15 minutes. Add the peas and return to the oven for a further 10–15 minutes or until the rice is tender and has absorbed the cooking liquid and the chicken is cooked through. Add a little more hot stock if the mixture is too dry.

6 Serve straight from the casserole with extra green vegetables.

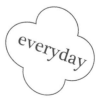

everyday

chicken korma

A tasty alternative to fat- and salt-laden takeaways.

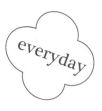
everyday

serves 4

2 tbsp olive oil

2 medium onions, peeled
and chopped

2 garlic cloves, peeled
and crushed

1 medium apple, peeled
and chopped

4 tsp mild curry powder

450g (1lb) skinless, boneless
chicken breasts, cut into
bite-size chunks

300ml (10fl oz/1¼ cups) hot
chicken stock

25g (1oz/⅛ cup) sultanas
(golden raisins)

2 tbsp tomato purée (paste)

125g (4½oz/⅔ cup)
basmati rice

sprinkling of chopped fresh
coriander (cilantro),
plus sprigs of coriander
to garnish

8 tbsp low-fat crème fraîche
or fromage frais

freshly ground black pepper

1 Over a medium heat, heat the olive oil in a large saucepan and sauté the onions, garlic and apple for 3–4 minutes, then stir in the curry powder.

2 Add the chunks of chicken and cook, stirring continuously for 2–3 minutes, until sealed all over.

3 Next add the hot chicken stock, sultanas (golden raisins), and tomato purée (paste) and bring to the boil. Reduce the heat to low, cover and simmer gently for about 30 minutes.

4 Twelve minutes before the end of cooking time, put the rice on to cook in a large saucepan, following the packet instructions.

5 Just before serving, add the chopped coriander (cilantro) and 4 tablespoons of low-fat crème fraîche or fromage frais to the curry and stir in well. Season with freshly ground black pepper and cook for a further 2 minutes but DO NOT boil.

6 Serve the curry with the hot cooked rice, adding one tablespoon of crème fraîche to each portion as you serve. Garnish with sprigs of coriander (cilantro).

Tip:

Some curry spices are thought to ease common ailments: turmeric is believed to help digestion; ginger may soothe coughs and colds and clear the head; garlic may help to treat inflamed skin; peppercorns could help with digestion and relieve constipation; and cumin is said to help flatulence and chesty coughs. So curries can be very healthy!

spicy chicken with red cabbage and beetroot

This tasty dish proves that low-fat and healthy does not mean boring. If you don't like things too spicy, just omit the paprika. The perfect accompaniment to this is a side dish of vitamin-rich new potatoes.

serves 4

4 skinless, boneless chicken breast fillets

1 tsp paprika

4 tbsp olive oil

1 red onion, peeled and finely sliced

400g (14oz) red cabbage, finely shredded

1 tsp dried chilli flakes (red pepper flakes)

250g (9oz) beetroot, trimmed and cut into matchsticks

1 small handful of chopped fresh flat-leaf parsley, to serve

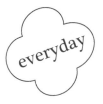

1 Dust the chicken fillets with the paprika.

2 Heat 2 tablespoons of the olive oil in a large frying pan set over a low to medium heat and add the chicken pieces. Fry them for 20 minutes, turning halfway through, until thoroughly cooked.

3 Meanwhile, heat the remaining oil in a large lidded saucepan and fry the onion for about 5 minutes until it starts to brown and soften. Add the cabbage and chilli flakes, and cook for a further 5 minutes, stirring occasionally.

4 Add the beetroot and cover. Cook gently for about 10 minutes until the vegetables have softened but still retain a little bite.

5 Remove the cabbage mixture to warmed serving plates. Sprinkle with the chopped parsley and place the chicken pieces on top. Now quickly add 1 tablespoon of water to the pan and heat through, taking in all the red juices left over from the beetroot and other veg. Pour this over the chicken and serve.

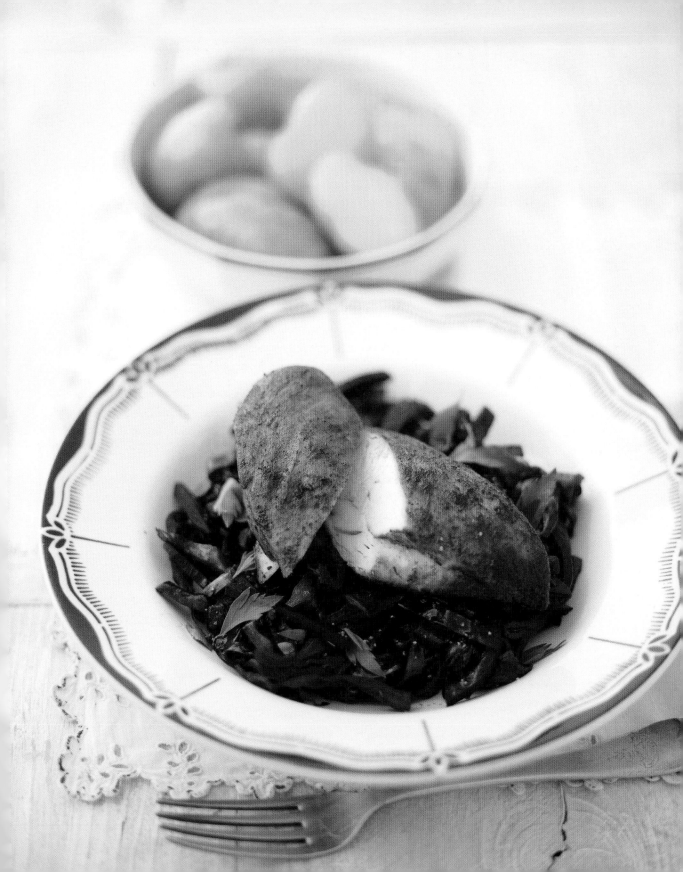

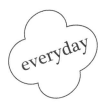

healthy chinese chicken wraps

I love the convenience of wraps but all the shop-bought ones are quite high in salt and fat. This dish gives you all the excitement of Chinese food and also, the feeling of a wrap, but because you use iceberg lettuce leaves instead of the wrap, it is still an everyday dish that can be enjoyed again and again.

serves 4

2 tbsp rice wine vinegar

2 tbsp reduced salt soy sauce

zest of 1 lemon

2 tbsp caster sugar

1 pinch of dried chilli flakes (red pepper flakes)

1 tsp freshly ground black pepper

1 iceberg lettuce

1 tbsp olive oil

1 bunch of spring onions (scallions), sliced thinly on the diagonal

4 carrots, peeled and cut into matchsticks

4 small skinless, boneless chicken breasts, very thinly sliced

2 garlic cloves, peeled and finely chopped

2.5cm (1in) fresh ginger, peeled and grated

2 tbsp finely chopped fresh coriander (cilantro)

1 In a bowl, mix together the rice wine vinegar, soy sauce, lemon zest, sugar, chilli flakes (red pepper flakes) and freshly ground black pepper, then set aside.

2 Separate the lettuce leaves, wash well, dry and place on a large platter. Set aside.

3 In a large frying pan set over a medium heat, heat the olive oil and cook the spring onions (scallions) for 2 minutes until they start to soften. Add the carrots and chicken and stir-fry until the chicken is cooked through (this should take a maximum of 4 minutes if the chicken is sliced very finely).

4 Stir in the garlic and ginger and cook, stirring continuously for 1–2 minutes, ensuring the chicken is well coated with all of the juices from the pan. Then pour over the rice wine mixture and continue to cook for another 2 minutes.

5 Spoon the stir-fry into a large serving bowl and sprinkle over the coriander (cilantro).

6 Let everyone help themselves and build their own wraps by spooning some of the chicken mixture into a lettuce leaf and folding the edges of leaf in to form delicious a little parcel.

spicy chicken kebabs

Better than a takeaway, this dish is a family favourite. Serve it with a large green salad and wholemeal pitta bread to make it a feast. This is an affordable, nutritious and fun meal to eat.

serves 4

2 tbsp olive oil

1 handful of fresh flat-leaf parsley

1 small bunch of chives

2 garlic cloves, peeled

½ tsp paprika

1 tsp ground cumin

zest and juice of 1 lemon

4 skinless chicken breasts, cut into bite-size chunks

1 red (bell) pepper, deseeded and cut into large chunks

1 green (bell) pepper, deseeded and cut into large chunks

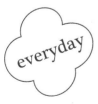

1 Leave 4–8 wooden skewers in a bowl of water to soak (this will prevent them from burning under the grill/broiler).

2 Put the olive oil in a blender, add the parsley (put in the entire stems), chives, garlic, paprika, cumin and lemon zest and juice and whiz to a paste.

3 Put the chicken into a medium-sized bowl and add the spicy paste. Give the chicken a good stir to ensure that it is all coated well. Pop in the refrigerator to marinate for about 20 minutes. (You can prepare this part of the recipe ahead of time if you like, and leave the chicken in the refrigerator to marinate overnight.)

4 Preheat the grill (broiler) to high. Thread the marinated chicken and (bell) peppers alternately onto presoaked skewers and grill (broil) for 10–12 minutes, turning occasionally, until the meat is cooked through.

5 Serve with a salad and wholemeal pitta bread. Have extra portions of lemon on the table to squeeze over for extra zing!

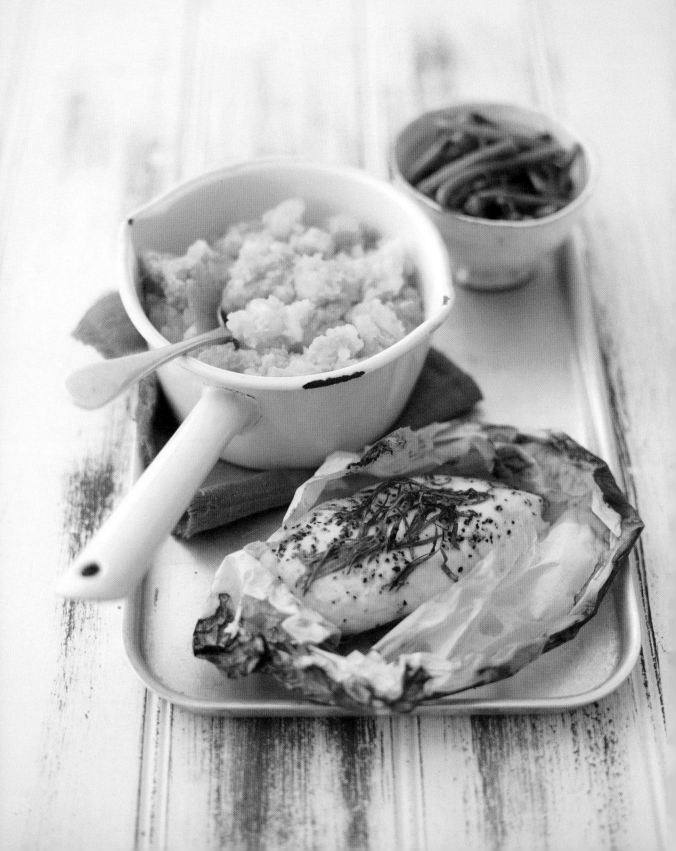

tarragon chicken with celeriac mash

In this gently flavoured chicken dish, the mash is made with a mixture of celeriac and sweet potato and doesn't need any butter added to it. Together with a good helping of green vegetables, this makes a highly nutritious meal.

serves 4

800g (1¾lb) sweet potatoes, peeled and chopped

200g (7oz) celeriac (celery root), peeled and chopped

4 skinless, boneless chicken breasts

8 sprigs of fresh tarragon

8 tbsp white wine

freshly ground black pepper

knob of butter

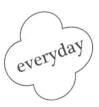
everyday

1 Preheat the oven to 200°C/400°F/Gas mark 6.

2 Cook the sweet potatoes and celeriac together in a large pan of boiling water for about 20 minutes or until tender.

3 Meanwhile, place the chicken breasts on a large piece of baking parchment or kitchen foil. Add 2 sprigs of tarragon on each, then sprinkle each with 2 tablespoons of white wine and some freshly ground black pepper. Place a little of the butter on each piece of chicken. Fold the paper to enclose the chicken and liquid completely and place in a roasting tin.

4 Cook the chicken in the centre of the oven for 25 minutes or until the juices run clear when it is pierced with a skewer.

5 When the potatoes and celeriac are cooked, drain them and mash together with some freshly ground black pepper. (You can add a dash of skimmed milk if the mash is a little dry.)

6 Serve the chicken on top of the mash and pour over any juice from the baking parchment parcel. Accompany it with a big portion of your favourite veggies and some yummy chicken gravy.

chicken in garlic sauce

Simple, clean flavours at their best. Don't be put off by the large quantity of garlic in this recipe – the cooking method gives the chicken a very gentle garlic infusion – and the alcohol in the cider burns off during cooking. Although this dish is traditionally made using double cream, I have substituted low-fat crème fraîche, which works a dream. This is delicious served with a portion of rice and broccoli for a nutritionally balanced, filling meal.

serves 4

15 garlic cloves, unpeeled

2 tbsp olive oil

4 skinless, boneless chicken breasts

1 bay leaf

450ml (16fl oz/2 cups) dry cider

200ml (7fl oz/¾ cup) apple juice

200ml (7fl oz/¾ cup) low-fat crème fraîche

freshly ground black pepper

1 tbsp fresh thyme leaves

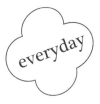
everyday

1 Preheat the oven to 180°C/350°F/Gas mark 4.

2 In a small pan set over a high heat, cook the whole, unpeeled garlic cloves in boiling water for 4 minutes. Drain, cool slightly, then peel and set aside.

3 Next, heat the olive oil in an ovenproof lidded casserole dish. Add the chicken and cook for 3–4 minutes on each side, or until turning brown.

4 Now add the blanched garlic cloves, bay leaf, cider and apple juice. Cover and transfer to the oven for 20–25 minutes, or until the chicken is cooked through.

5 When cooked, lift the chicken out of the casserole dish and keep warm. Remove half the garlic cloves and discard. Now, on the hob, bring the casserole juices to the boil. Crush the garlic into the juices with a fork, then reduce the heat and simmer until the sauce is reduced and thickened slightly.

6 Finally, add the low-fat crème fraîche, season with freshly ground black pepper and simmer for 1 minute. Return the chicken to the sauce and baste with the juices, then add the thyme leaves, give it one last stir and serve.

grilled tandoori chicken, cucumber & spring onion noodles

Please try to stay away from salt- and fat-laden takeaways. They are expensive and will do your health no favours at all. Follow this very easy recipe for a much healthier alternative and you'll never turn back!

serves 4

4 chicken breasts

300g (10oz/1¼ cups) fat-free thick plain yogurt

juice of 1 lemon

½ onion, peeled and finely chopped

1 garlic clove, peeled and crushed

1 tsp grated fresh ginger

2 tsp garam masala

1 tsp cayenne pepper

8 spring onions (scallions)

1 cucumber

2 tsp finely chopped fresh coriander (cilantro) leaves

1 lemon, cut into wedges

1 lime, cut into wedges

1 Prepare the chicken by cutting slits in the breasts lengthways. Put them in a shallow dish.

2 In another bowl, mix together the fat-free yogurt, lemon juice, onion, garlic, ginger, garam masala and cayenne pepper. Mix until smooth, then spread mixture over the chicken breasts. Cover and refrigerate for as long as you can. A couple of hours will do but overnight would be even better.

3 To cook, either barbecue on an outdoor grill, or if the weather won't allow, grill (broil) under a high heat for 6–8 minutes on each side, ensuring the chicken is cooked through and that, when pierced with a skewer, the juices run clear.

4 Meanwhile, trim the spring onions (scallions) and the cucumber and, using a potato peeler, shave strips lengthways to create long, flat 'noodles'.

5 Serve the chicken on top of the noodles and garnish with the chopped coriander (cilantro) leaves and lemon and lime wedges.

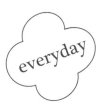
everyday

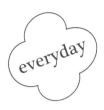

chinese chicken with lots of veggies

There are so many ways to cook chicken. Stir-frying marinated chicken is one of the quickest ways and goes well with pretty much any vegetable. Feel free to swap the veggies around for those that are in season, more affordable or simply left over in your refrigerator.

serves 2

4 skinless, boneless chicken breasts

50g (2oz) mangetout (snow peas)

50g (2oz) baby sweetcorn (corn)

50g (2oz) button (white) mushrooms

50g (2oz) French (green) beans

2 tbsp olive oil

1 red (bell) pepper, deseeded and cut into strips

1 tbsp sesame seeds

for the marinade

1 small garlic clove, peeled and crushed

1cm (½in) fresh ginger, peeled and grated

3 tbsp soy sauce

½ tbsp clear honey

½ tbsp wine vinegar or sherry

1 large pinch of turmeric

1 tbsp tomato purée (paste)

1 Start by mixing all the marinade ingredients together in a bowl. Set aside.

2 Cut the chicken into the thinnest strips you possibly can. I find it easiest to work with frozen chicken just as it is starting to defrost. With a really sharp knife, you can cut really fine strips from the chicken. It will then defrost very quickly once cut.

3 Mix the chicken with the marinade, cover and leave for about an hour in the refrigerator.

4 Meanwhile, blanch the mangetout (snow peas), baby sweetcorn (corn), button mushrooms and French beans by dropping into boiling water for 2 minutes, then refresh in ice-cold water and set aside.

5 Heat the olive oil in a wok, add the chicken and red (bell) peppers and stir-fry with the marinade until the chicken is firm – this will take 4–5 minutes. Then add the blanched vegetables and, when thoroughly heated though, pile onto a warmed serving dish and sprinkle with the sesame seeds.

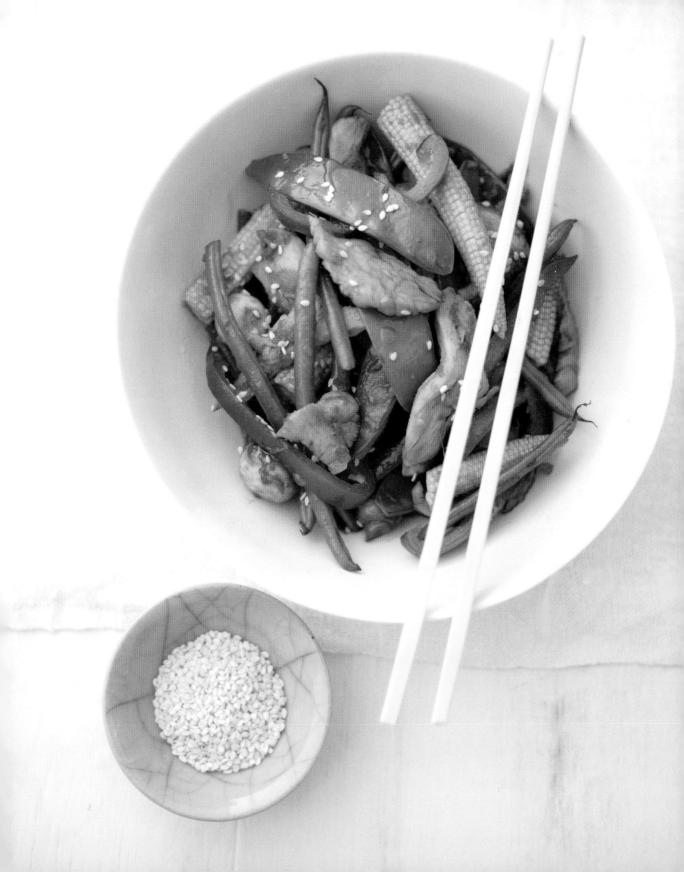

quick-grilled chicken with mango salsa

If you are in a hurry for lunch but don't want to sacrifice great taste and nutrition, give this delicious chicken dish a go. It's very, very quick and easy to make, but it'll give your taste buds a party!

serves 4

4 skinless, boneless chicken breasts
2 tbsp olive oil
juice of 1 lime
freshly ground black pepper
1 large tomato, diced
2 spring onions (scallions), diced
1 mango, diced
1 small fennel bulb, trimmed and diced
1 fresh red or green chilli, deseeded and finely chopped
2 tbsp balsamic vinegar
2 tbsp chopped fresh flat-leaf parsley
2 tbsp fresh chopped mint
baby spinach and watercress salad leaves, to serve

1 Before you start cooking the chicken, take all the fruit out of the refrigerator and bring to room temperature (much tastier than serving cold).

2 Preheat the grill (broiler) to medium.

3 Put the chicken on a grill (broiler) pan and drizzle over 1 tablespoon of olive oil and half the lime juice, then sprinkle with freshly ground black pepper. Grill (broil) for 8–10 minutes on each side or until the chicken is cooked through and the juices run clear when it is pierced with a skewer. Set aside.

4 In a large bowl, mix the remaining ingredients and season with freshly ground black pepper. Spoon on top of the chicken and serve with spinach and watercress salad.

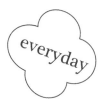
everyday

spicy, easy chicken tagine

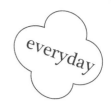
everyday

The easiest, tastiest dish from a foreign land. Enjoy this all year round with friends, family, or indulgently alone.

serves 4

2 tbsp olive oil

1 red onion, peeled and chopped

2 garlic cloves, peeled and crushed

2.5cm (1in) fresh ginger, peeled and grated

1 tsp ground cumin

1 tsp paprika

1 tsp chilli powder

4 skinless, boneless chicken breasts, cubed

1 x 400g (14oz) tin chopped tomatoes

1 cinnamon stick

1 small butternut squash, peeled and cubed

75g (3oz/½ cup) raisins

300ml (10fl oz/1¼ cups) chicken stock

1 In a large lidded tagine or non-stick saucepan, heat the olive oil over a medium heat and add the onion, garlic and ginger. Fry for 3–4 minutes until starting to colour.

2 Now add the cumin, paprika and chilli powder and fry for another minute.

3 Next add the chicken. Increase the heat to high to quickly brown and seal the chicken.

4 Reduce the heat to medium and add all the remaining ingredients, cover and simmer gently for an hour. Serve with nutty wholemeal (wholewheat) bread to mop up the delicious juices!

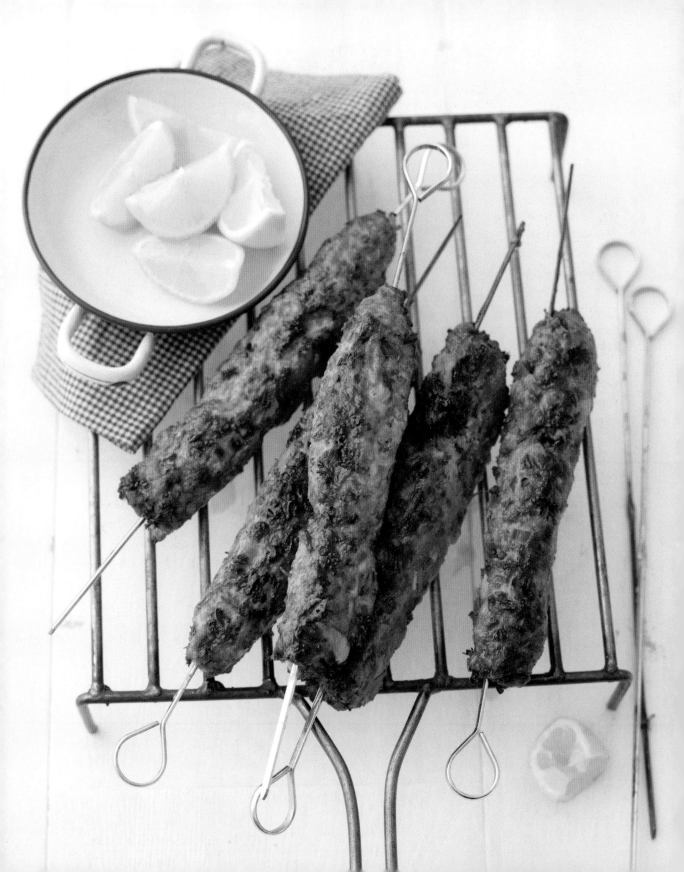

lemony turkey kebabs

Fresh lemons and lemon thyme bring a wonderfully zingy flavour to this lovely summery delight.

makes 6–8

1kg (2lb 2oz) turkey mince (ground turkey)

1 handful of fresh lemon thyme leaves, chopped

1 handful of fresh curly parsley, chopped

2 garlic cloves, peeled and crushed

2 shallots, peeled and finely diced

½ red (bell) pepper, deseeded and finely diced

½ red chilli, deseeded and finely diced (optional)

1 egg

zest of 1 lemon

freshly ground black pepper

lemon wedges, to serve

1 Light your barbecue, preheat the grill (broiler) to its highest setting or prepare your griddle pan on your hob.

2 In a large bowl, bind together the minced (ground) turkey, chopped herbs, crushed garlic and the diced shallots, (bell) pepper and red chilli (if using) with the egg and lemon zest. I find this is a job best done with your hands. Season with freshly ground black pepper.

3 Once thoroughly mixed together, take a small handful and shape around a metal or presoaked wooden skewer (see p81), compacting the mixture well and making a long 'shish' or sausage shape. (If you don't have any skewers to hand you can always make this mixture into a patty or burger shape.)

4 As you finish each kebab, put it straight on to the barbecue. Cook for 8–10 minutes, turning when required. Be careful not to turn them too soon or they might fall apart. Ensure the meat is cooked all the way through before serving with lemon wedges.

Tip:

Metal skewers speed up the cooking time because, as they heat up, they help to cook the inside of the kebabs.

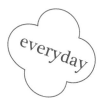

everyday

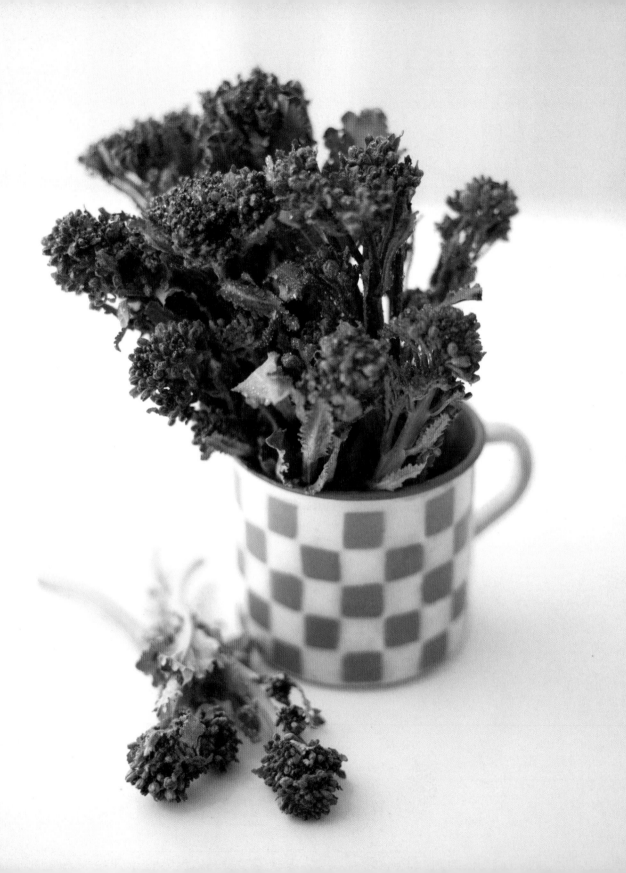

fish

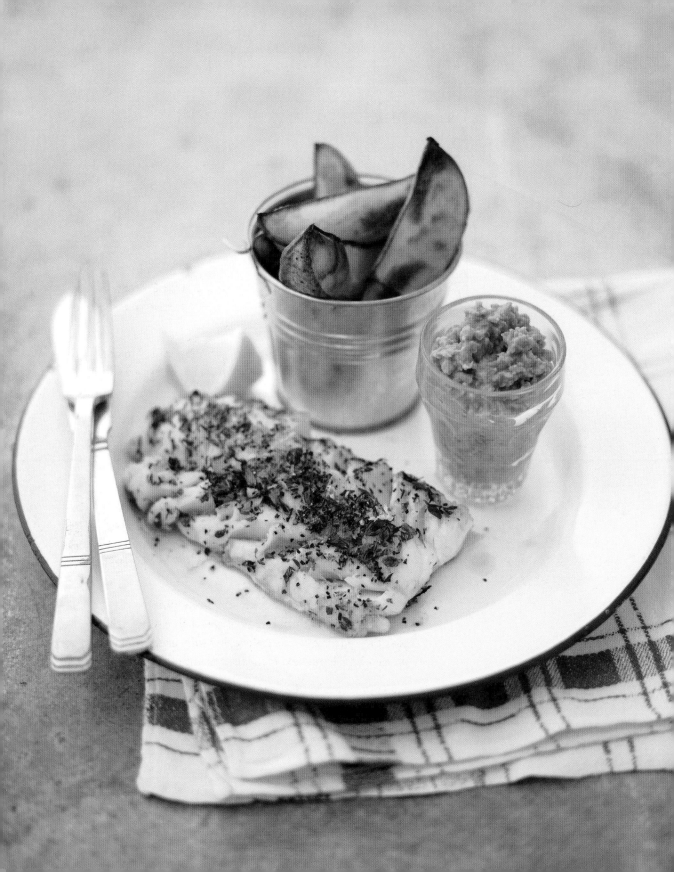

healthy fish, chips and mushy peas

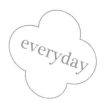
everyday

Yippee – healthy fish, chips and mushy peas ... what more can I say? Except that potatoes cooked in this way are full of nutrients, and peas are a wonderful source of vitamin C, protein, fibre and folate.

serves 2

450g (1lb) large organic potatoes, washed and cut into slim wedges (if you don't have organic, ensure you peel the potatoes)

3 tbsp olive oil

2 x 200g (7oz) thick cod or haddock fillets

2 tbsp chopped fresh lemon thyme leaves

freshly ground black pepper

zest of 1 lemon

350g (12oz/3 cups) frozen peas

2 tbsp low-fat crème fraîche

2 tbsp chopped fresh mint

squeeze of lemon juice

lemon wedges, to serve

1 Preheat oven to 200°C/400°F/Gas mark 6.

2 Put the prepared potato wedges into a large bowl and add 2 tablespoons of olive oil. Mix well so that all the potatoes are glistening in the oil.

3 If you have one, put a wire rack over a roasting tin and arrange the potato wedges on top. Pop into the oven and cook for 30–35 minutes.

4 Meanwhile, drizzle the remaining olive oil over the fish fillets and sprinkle on the chopped lemon thyme, some freshly ground black pepper and the lemon zest. Rub them in with your hands on both sides of the fish.

5 In a large frying pan set over a medium heat, cook the fish on both sides for just 2 minutes per fillet to seal in the flavours. Then transfer the fish to a baking tray and cook in the oven for about 15 minutes until it is tender and flaking.

6 Meanwhile, cook the peas in boiling water for 8–10 minutes until very tender. Drain well, return to the pan, then add the crème fraîche and mint and whiz to a purée with a hand-held blender until almost smooth.

7 Season the mushy peas and fish with freshly ground black pepper and a squeeze of lemon and serve with the chips on the side and lemon wedges.

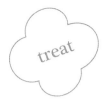
treat

smoked haddock and leek pie

I've marked this dish as a treat because it contains some cheese and milk – although this is a great recipe that is relatively low in fat compared to the usual fish pie recipes. Always use un-dyed smoked haddock. This can easily be doubled or halved if you want to make less or more!

serves 4

1 tsp olive oil

1 onion, peeled and finely chopped

2 leeks, trimmed and finely chopped

150g (5oz/1⅓ cups) spinach

150g (5oz/1⅓ cups) frozen peas

450g (1lb) undyed smoked haddock fillet

300ml (10fl oz/1¼ cups) skimmed milk

1 tbsp plain (all-purpose) flour

50g (2oz) low-fat mature Cheddar cheese, grated

freshly ground black pepper

3 slices wholemeal (wholewheat) bread, whizzed in a food processor to make breadcrumbs

1 Preheat the oven to 200°C/400°F/Gas mark 6.

2 In a large lidded saucepan set over a medium heat, heat the olive oil, add the onion with 2 tablespoons of water and fry for about 10 minutes until soft. Next add the leeks, spinach and frozen peas, cover and cook for 5 minutes. Take off the heat and set aside.

3 Take another large saucepan and add the fish and milk. Bring to the boil, then turn off the heat straight away. Remove the fish (reserve the milk) and put it into a 1.5 litre (2½ pint/1.5 quart) shallow ovenproof dish. Using 2 forks, gently break up the fish. Now add the onion-and-leek mixture.

4 Next, take a small ladleful of the reserved milk, put it into a pan and whisk in the flour. Set the pan over a low heat and gradually add the remaining milk, whisking all the time, until the sauce simmers and thickens. Stir in half the cheese, season with freshly ground black pepper, then pour the sauce over the vegetables in the ovenproof dish.

5 Mix the breadcrumbs and remaining cheese in a bowl and sprinkle the mixture over the sauce.

6 Cook the pie in the oven for 25–30 minutes until bubbling, then serve immediately.

chilli prawns
with creamy basil sauce

This is a delicious low-fat treat. Prawns do contain some cholesterol so limit them to once a week and keep the portions small. Serve this with a large spinach and watercress salad for a nutritionally light lunch or starter.

serves 4

for the prawns

1 tbsp olive oil

1 garlic clove, peeled and
finely chopped

1 red chilli, deseeded and
finely chopped

20 raw tiger (jumbo shrimp)
prawns, peeled but tails
left on

2 tbsp balsamic vinegar

freshly ground black pepper

for the creamy sauce

4 tbsp low-fat fromage frais

juice of ½ lemon

½ tsp Dijon mustard

2 tbsp olive oil

1 large handful of fresh
basil leaves, chopped very
finely or whizzed in a
small food processor

1 Start by making the sauce. Simply put all the sauce ingredients into a bowl and mix together. Set aside.

2 To cook the prawns, heat the olive oil in a large frying pan set over a fairly high heat. Add the chopped garlic and chilli and sauté for 1 minute, stirring occasionally. Tip the prawns and the balsamic vinegar into the pan and cook for 3–4 minutes until the prawns turn pink. Season with freshly ground black pepper.

3 Serve immediately, with the creamy basil sauce on the side.

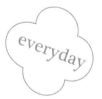

everyday

cod with pesto topping and butter bean mash

With protein from the fish, fibre from the beans and vitamins and iron from the spinach, this delicious dish is a winner!

serves 4

4 unsmoked cod fillets

4 tbsp shop-bought red pesto

2 tbsp olive oil

2 x 410g (14oz) tins butter (lima) beans, drained and rinsed

2 garlic cloves, peeled and crushed

250g (9oz) spinach

8 capers in brine, rinsed and drained

2 lemons, cut into wedges, to serve

freshly ground black pepper

1 Preheat the grill (broiler) to medium.

2 Arrange the cod fillets on a baking tray that will fit under your grill. Spread 1 tablespoon of red pesto over each of the cod fillets and grill (broil) them for 10–15 minutes until the flesh is opaque and just cooked.

3 Meanwhile, heat the olive oil in a large frying set over a medium heat and add the drained butter (lima) beans and garlic. Cook for 10 minutes, stirring occasionally and mashing the beans lightly with a fork as you go. You are not aiming for a smooth mash consistency, rather a crushed bean consistency.

4 About 2 minutes before serving, add the spinach and capers to the pan and allow the spinach to wilt. Spoon the butter bean mash on to warmed plates and top with the cod and any juices.

5 Serve with a squeeze of lemon over each fish fillet and season with plenty of freshly ground black pepper.

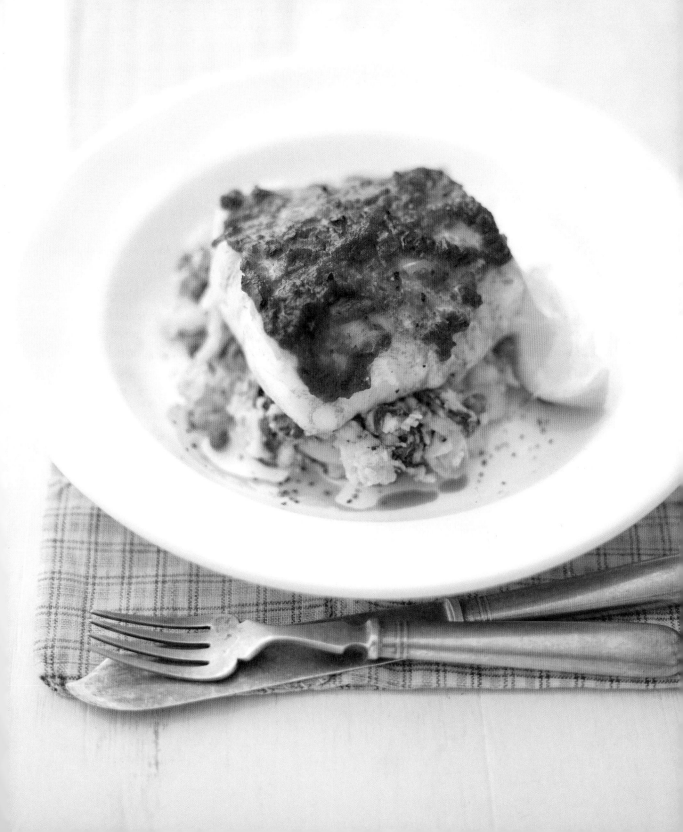

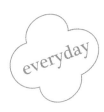

salmon and asparagus pasta

This quick and easy dish is marked as a treat because it contains some low-fat soft cheese. If you crave the calorie-laden cheesy sauces, give this one a try. It's nice and light yet will satisfy your craving in a much healthier way. Try to use wholewheat pasta – this will fill you up more, which means you won't need such a big portion.

serves 2

100g (3½oz) asparagus
　spears
2 tbsp olive oil
1 garlic clove, peeled and
　finely chopped
¼ teaspoon dried chilli
　flakes (red pepper flakes)
150g (5oz) fresh salmon fillet
110g (4oz) dried wholewheat
　pasta of your choice
juice of ½ lemon
100g (3½oz/½ cup) low-fat
　soft cheese
2 tbsp chopped fresh dill
freshly ground black pepper

1 Snap off the woody ends of the asparagus and cut each stalk on the diagonal into 2.5cm (1in) pieces.

2 Heat the olive oil in a non-stick frying pan set over a medium–high heat. Add the garlic and dried chilli flakes and sauté for 30 seconds. Add the salmon fillet and cook for 3 minutes on each side. Take off the heat and set aside.

3 Meanwhile, cook the pasta according to the packet instructions, adding the asparagus 3 minutes before the end of the cooking time. Drain well, return to the saucepan and add the lemon juice and low-fat soft cheese. Stir over a low heat for 1 minute.

4 Prepare the salmon by removing any skin and bones and cut it into bite-size pieces. Add it to the pasta, toss gently and serve sprinkled with dill and freshly ground black pepper.

chinese five-spice salmon

Five spice is great to keep in your store cupboard. It is a blend of star anise, fennel, cinnamon, cloves and peppercorns and is used in many traditional Chinese dishes. If you love Chinese takeaways but want a healthier option, this delicious dish is packed with goodness that has an authentic Chinese flavour without any of the naughties!

serves 4

2 tsp Chinese five spice

4 salmon fillets, each weighing about 125g (4½oz), skinned

freshly ground black pepper

4 spring onions (scallions), cut lengthways into thin strips

1 large leek, cut lengthways into thin strips

1 large carrot, peeled, trimmed and cut lengthways into thin strips

115g (4oz) mangetout (snow peas), shredded and cut lengthways into thin strips

2.5cm (1in) fresh ginger, finely sliced

2 tbsp white wine

1 tbsp low-salt soy sauce or lemon juice

1 tbsp olive oil, plus extra for drizzling

1 Rub the five spice powder into both sides of the fish fillets and season with freshly ground black pepper. Set aside.

2 Preheat the grill (broiler) to medium.

3 Put the spring onions (scallions), leek, carrot and mangetout (snow peas) into a large bowl. Add the ginger, white wine and soy sauce or lemon juice. Mix well.

4 Put the salmon fillets on the grill (broiler) rack and sprinkle with freshly ground black pepper and a little drizzle of olive oil. Grill (broil) for 3–4 minutes on each side until cooked through.

5 While the salmon is cooking, heat 1 tablespoon of oil in a preheated wok or large heavy-based frying pan and stir-fry the vegetables for 4–5 minutes until just tender. Remember that the vegetables are all finely sliced, so won't take long to cook.

6 Transfer the vegetables to serving plates and serve with the salmon on top.

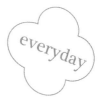
everyday

simply marinated tuna

This is a simple dish both in method and flavour. If you are happy with a little spice, leave the chillies in; if you prefer a calmer dish, leave them out – no problem. Serve with fresh new potatoes and a green salad.

serves 4

4 shallots, peeled and
  finely sliced

zest and juice of 4 lemons

4 capers in brine, rinsed
  and drained

3 tbsp olive oil

1 red or green chilli,
  deseeded and diced

freshly ground black pepper

4 x 125g (4½oz) tuna fillets,
  thinly sliced

1 In a large bowl, mix together the shallots, lemon juice and zest, capers, olive oil, chilli and freshly ground black pepper. Add the sliced tuna, cover the bowl and leave in the refrigerator to marinate for 12 hours, turning occasionally.

2 When ready to cook, heat a grill (broiler) or barbecue to hot. Take the tuna from the marinade and cook the fish for 1–2 minutes on each side for rare, or for 4 minutes for well done, and serve at once, drizzled with the remaining marinade.

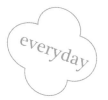

everyday

crusty herby haddock

The herby crust makes this haddock particularly tempting...

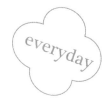

everyday

serves 4

1 tbsp olive oil, plus extra
   for oiling

4 x 140g (4¾oz) unsmoked,
   undyed haddock fillets

20 cherry tomatoes (stalks
   left on)

100g (3½oz/2 cups)
   wholemeal (wholewheat)
   breadcrumbs (you'll need
   about 4 slices of bread)

1 garlic clove, peeled and
   crushed

zest and juice of 1 lemon

2 handfuls of fresh flat-leaf
   parsley, chopped

freshly ground black pepper

1 Preheat the oven to 200°C/400°F/Gas mark 6.

2 Lightly oil a baking tray with olive oil, then arrange the
   haddock fillets and cherry tomatoes (stalks left on) on
   the baking tray. Set aside.

3 In a large bowl, mix together the breadcrumbs, garlic,
   lemon zest and juice, olive oil, parsley and freshly
   ground black pepper. Divide this mixture between the
   4 haddock fillets, patting it on to the top of each fillet,
   then bake for about 15 minutes or until the fish flakes
   slightly and the topping has gone nice and crusty.

4 Serve with a big side salad for a delicious lunch or light
   evening meal.

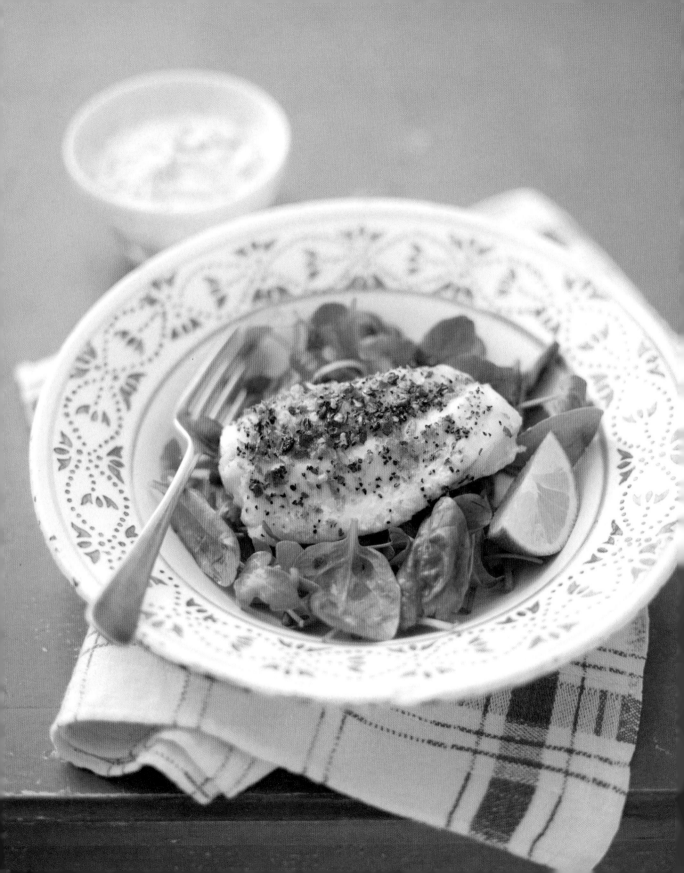

roast monkfish
with olives and capers

I absolutely adore monkfish (it's a very ugly fish but totally delicious). In this super-quick and easy recipe the monkfish is nicely filling and the sauce lovely and light.

serves 4

4 x 175g (6oz) monkfish
 fillets

zest and juice of 1 lime

1 garlic clove, peeled and
 finely chopped

1 tbsp olive oil

1 small pinch of dried chilli
 flakes (red pepper flakes),
 plus extra for sprinkling

freshly ground black pepper

4 tbsp low-fat natural yogurt

25g (1oz) pitted black olives,
 roughly chopped

1 tbsp capers, rinsed
 and chopped

2 tbsp chopped fresh parsley

lime wedges, to serve

1 Preheat the oven to 190°C/375°F/Gas mark 5.

2 Prepare the monkfish by pulling away any whitish
 membrane from the flesh. Place in a roasting tin
 and sprinkle with the lime zest and juice, garlic,
 olive oil, dried chilli flakes (red pepper flakes) and
 black pepper. Roast for 20 minutes until the fish is
 cooked through.

3 Meanwhile, mix together the yogurt, olives, capers and
 parsley and season with freshly ground black pepper
 to taste.

4 Serve the fish with the dressing on the side, sprinkled
 with a few dried chilli flakes (red pepper flakes), and
 accompanied with a big green salad and lime wedges
 to serve.

everyday

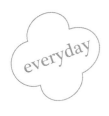

grilled mackerel with cherry tomatoes

Mackerel is a super-healthy oily fish and it works really well with sweet cherry tomatoes.

serves 4

4 fresh mackerel (ask
  your fishmonger to
  clean them)

freshly ground black pepper

3 tbsp olive oil

1 red onion, peeled
  and chopped

1 garlic clove, peeled
  and chopped

1 x 400g (14oz) tin chopped
  tomatoes

1 tsp caster sugar

1 sweet pointed red (bell)
  pepper, chopped

125g (4½oz) cherry
  tomatoes, cut in half

3 tbsp red wine vinegar

4 tbsp chopped fresh basil,
  plus some basil leaves,
  to garnish

lemon wedges, to serve

1 Slash the mackerel 2–3 times on each side and season
  with freshly ground black pepper. Put on a grill
  (broiler) rack and set aside.

2 Heat 1 tablespoon of the olive oil in a large saucepan and
  cook the onion and garlic for 5 minutes until softened.

3 Now add the tinned tomatoes, sugar and red (bell)
  pepper. Bring to the boil and reduce the heat to simmer
  for 10 minutes until reduced and thickened. Add the
  cherry tomatoes and simmer for another 5 minutes.

4 Next, make the basil vinaigrette. Put the red wine
  vinegar into a bowl with the remaining 2 tablespoons
  of olive oil, the chopped basil and some more freshly
  ground black pepper. Whisk well together and set aside.

5 Preheat the grill (broiler) to high and grill (broil) the
  mackerel for 4–5 minutes on each side until cooked.

6 Finally, stir the basil vinaigrette into the reduced
  tomato mixture. Put the mackerel on to four warmed
  serving plates. Spoon over the tomato mixture
  and garnish with fresh basil leaves. Serve with
  lemon wedges.

fish in white wine with fennel

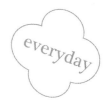
everyday

Fennel is great for the digestive system and gives the cod a lovely flavour in this recipe. Eat the fish alone or serve up with new potatoes or brown rice, and with lots of green veggies.

serves 4

1 tbsp olive oil

2 medium red onions, peeled and finely sliced

2 garlic cloves, peeled and crushed

2 small or 1 large fennel bulb, trimmed and finely sliced

2 tbsp chopped fresh dill, plus extra for sprinkling

1 small glass white wine

4 x 150g (5oz) cod fillets

freshly ground black pepper

1 Preheat the oven to 200°C/400°F/Gas mark 6.

2 Heat the olive oil in a flameproof lidded casserole dish set over a medium heat. When sizzling, add the onions, garlic and fennel, then cover and cook, stirring occasionally, for 5 minutes or until the onions are soft and translucent.

3 Next, add the chopped dill and white wine and bring quickly to the boil.

4 Now sit the fish fillets on top of the fennel mixture, season well with freshly ground black pepper, then put the casserole in the oven and cook for 10 minutes, basting the fish occasionally with the juices.

4 Sprinkle with plenty of extra dill and serve immediately with new potatoes or brown rice and green veggies.

thai salmon fish cakes with wild rocket salad

A lovely and light yet filling dish. Feel free to miss out the Thai curry paste if you are not a fan.

serves 4

2 x 213g (7oz) tins red
    salmon, drained

1 tbsp Thai red curry paste

1 tbsp cornflour (cornstarch)

zest and juice of 2 limes

2 spring onions (scallions),
    finely chopped

2 tbsp frozen sweetcorn
    (corn), thawed

2 tbsp chopped fresh basil

1 egg, beaten

freshly ground black pepper

3 tbsp plain (all-purpose)
    flour

2 tbsp olive oil, plus a little
    extra for the salad

1 bag of wild rocket
    (arugula)

juice of 1 lemon

lime wedges, to serve

1 Flake the salmon and discard any skin and small bones. Put the fish in a bowl with the red curry paste, cornflour (cornstarch), lime zest and juice, spring onions (scallions), sweetcorn (corn), basil and egg. Season with black pepper and mix well. With wet hands, shape the mixture into 12 small fish cakes.

2 Put the plain (all-purpose) flour on to a plate and coat the fish cakes on both sides. Place them on a baking sheet. Cover and chill for 1 hour.

3 When ready to cook, heat the olive oil in a large non-stick frying pan and fry the fish cakes for 2–3 minutes on each side until golden.

4 Serve the fish cakes with wild rocket (arugula), lime wedges and drizzle over a little olive oil and lemon juice.

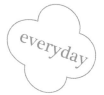

everyday

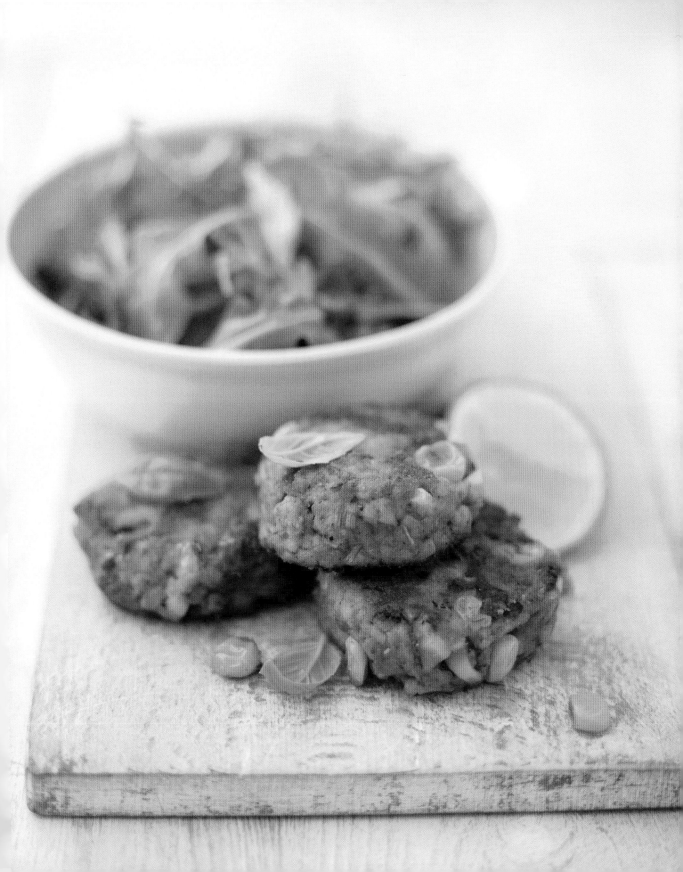

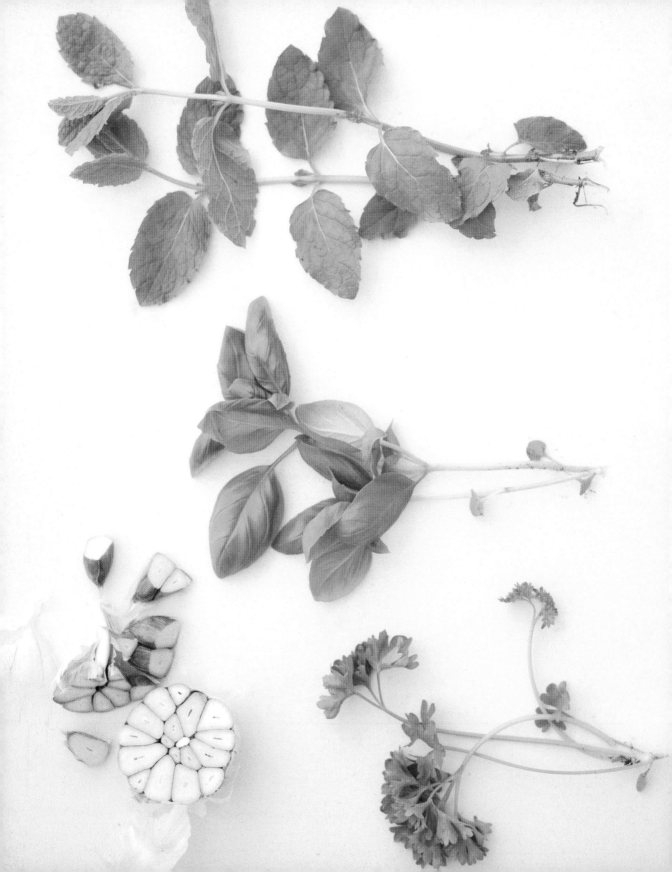

red meat

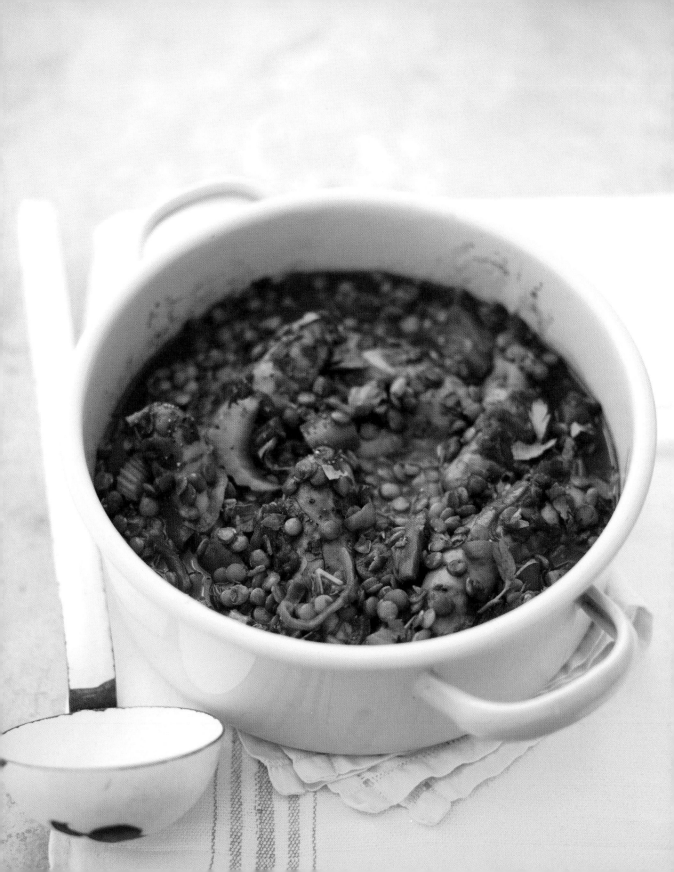

all-in-one lentil-and-sausage casserole

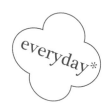

everyday*

Always try to buy best-quality sausages. I get mine from my local butcher who does a 'sin-free' sausage, which is made from 100 per cent meat. In this dish, lentils offer great fibre and, with the onions, garlic, olive oil and a small amount of red wine, create a deliciously heart-healthy meal.

serves 4–6

300g (10oz/1½ cups) green
  or brown lentils

6 pork sausages

2 tbsp olive oil

2 onions, peeled and sliced

3 celery sticks, chopped

2 garlic cloves, peeled
  and chopped

1 sweet pointed red (bell)
  pepper, diced

3 sprigs fresh thyme,
  leaves picked

1 bay leaf

3 large tomatoes, skinned
  and chopped

4 tbsp tomato purée (paste)

200ml (7fl oz/¾ cup)
  red wine

1 large bunch of fresh
  flat-leaf parsley, chopped

1 If you're using brown lentils, soak them overnight in cold water, then drain them and set aside.

2 Preheat the oven to 200°C/400°F/Gas mark 6.

3 Brown the sausages in a large lidded casserole dish set over a medium heat. Once they are nicely browned, remove from the dish and set them aside. Pour off any oil from the sausages and return the casserole dish to the hob.

4 Heat the olive oil in the same casserole dish. Add the onions, celery and garlic to the pan and sauté for 5 minutes.

5 Add the diced red (bell) pepper, thyme leaves, the bay leaf, tomatoes and tomato purée (paste), mix together and cook for 5 minutes, stirring regularly.

6 Add the lentils and red wine and give the mixture a good stir. Then add just enough water to cover all the ingredients – approximately 400ml (14fl oz/1¾ cup).

7 Place the sausages on top of the mixture, cover with the lid and cook in the oven for 30–40 minutes. Stir in the parsley just before serving.

* Although this dish is marked as an everyday dish, bear in mind that you should eat red meat no more than once a week.

spaghetti bolognese with extra vegetables

One of my family favourites, this dish has plenty of added nutrition, with all the extra veggies, but will still please your nostalgic streak!

serves 4

1 tbsp olive oil

1 onion, peeled and
   finely chopped

1 red (bell) pepper, finely
   chopped

1 green (bell) pepper, finely
   chopped

2 carrots, peeled and grated

2 garlic cloves, peeled
   and crushed

450g (1lb) extra-lean
   minced (ground) beef

4 tbsp tomato purée (paste)

300ml (10fl oz/1¼ cups) hot
   beef stock (a shop-bought
   cube is fine)

1 x 400g (14oz) tin chopped
   tomatoes

2 tbsp Worcestershire sauce

125g (4½oz) button (white)
   mushrooms, sliced

freshly ground black pepper

500g (1lb 2oz) dried
   spaghetti

1 Heat the olive oil in a large lidded non-stick pan set over a medium heat and fry the onion, diced peppers and grated carrots for 10 minutes until starting to soften. Add the garlic and cook for 1 minute.

2 Next, add the mince and brown evenly. Use a wooden spoon to break up the pieces. Now add the tomato purée and beef stock, cover and increase the heat a little.

3 When the stock starts to bubble, add the tomatoes, Worcestershire sauce, mushrooms and freshly ground black pepper to taste. Reduce the heat, cover and simmer, stirring occasionally, for 25 minutes.

4 A little while before the sauce has finished cooking, cook the pasta as per the packet instructions, timing it so that the pasta and sauce are ready at the same time. Drain the pasta well, return it to the pan and add the bolognese sauce. Toss to mix, check the seasoning, then tip into a serving dish and serve with a lovely green salad.

* Try to limit your consumption of red meat to once a week.

treat*

spanish pork-and-bean stew

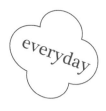
everyday

Another yummy dish to feed your body and soul. It offers loads of nutrition, is very filling, and I'm sure it will quickly become an everyday family meal.

serves 4

3 tbsp olive oil

400g (14oz) pork escalope
  (scallop), cut into 5cm
  (2in) cubes

1 onion, peeled and sliced

2 leeks, trimmed and cut
  into chunks

1 red (bell) pepper, deseeded
  and sliced

2 garlic cloves, peeled and
  crushed

2 celery sticks, cut into
  chunks

⅓ tsp cayenne pepper

3 tbsp tomato purée (paste)

1 x 400g (14oz) tin chopped
  tomatoes

300ml (10fl oz/1¼ cups) hot
  vegetable or chicken stock

freshly ground black pepper

1 x 400g (14oz) tin
  cannellini beans, drained
  and rinsed

1 tbsp chopped fresh parsley

1 lemon, quartered, to serve

low-fat crème fraîche,
  to serve

1 Preheat the oven to 180°C/350°F/Gas mark 4.

2 Heat 2 tablespoons of the olive oil in a large ovenproof casserole dish set over a medium heat and fry the pork in batches until golden. Remove the pork from the dish and set aside.

3 Heat the remaining olive oil in the casserole dish and fry the onion for 5–10 minutes until softened. Add the leeks, red (bell) pepper, garlic, celery and cayenne pepper and cook for 5 minutes. Return the pork to the casserole dish and add the tomato purée. Cook for 1–2 minutes, stirring constantly.

4 Now add the tomatoes and stock and season with freshly ground black pepper. Bring to the boil, then transfer the casserole dish to the oven and cook for 25 minutes.

5 Add the drained beans and return to the oven for 5 minutes to warm them through. Then stir in the parsley and serve with the lemon wedges and crème fraîche.

Tip:
This recipe traditionally uses pork, but you can also make it using chicken and turkey – all work equally well.

pork chops with apples and pears

I enjoy pork, especially with fruit. Of course, I advise cutting off all visible fat from your pork chops, but this lost flavour is more than compensated for with the delicious fruit and vegetables in this dish. Serve with rice or a baked sweet potato.

serves 4

4 pork loin chops

3 tbsp olive oil

1 tbsp fennel seeds, crushed

5cm (2in) fresh ginger, peeled and grated

450g (1lb) small parsnips, peeled and halved lengthways

200g (7oz) small leeks, trimmed and roughly sliced

2 Granny Smith apples, peeled, halved and cored

2 pears, peeled and halved

300ml (10fl oz/1¼ cups) apple juice

1 bay leaf

freshly ground black pepper

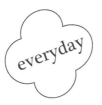

1 Preheat the oven to 200°C/400°F/Gas mark 6.

2 Cut off all visible fat from the pork chops. Rub the pork all over with 1 tablespoon of olive oil, the fennel seeds and ginger.

3 Heat the remaining olive oil in a large ovenproof casserole dish set over a medium heat. Cook the chops for 2 minutes on each side to brown them. Remove them and set aside.

4 Now put the parsnips into the casserole dish and stir until these are golden brown. Next, add the leeks, apples and pears, then sit the chops on top. Pour in half the apple juice, add the bay leaf and bake in the oven for about 30 minutes, depending on the thickness of the chops, turning everything occasionally during cooking so it colours evenly.

5 After 30 minutes, transfer the chops, parsnips, leeks, apple and pears to a serving dish, cover and keep warm. Put the casserole dish back on the hob over a high heat and stir in the remaining apple juice until it caramelises. Let it bubble, stirring in any tasty bits from the dish with a wooden spoon. Leave to bubble until the juice reduces to a syrupy liquid, then add seasoning and taste, adjusting the seasoning if necessary. Spoon this over the chops and fruit to serve.

6 Serve with a jacket potato, a baked sweet potato or rice. Yum yum!

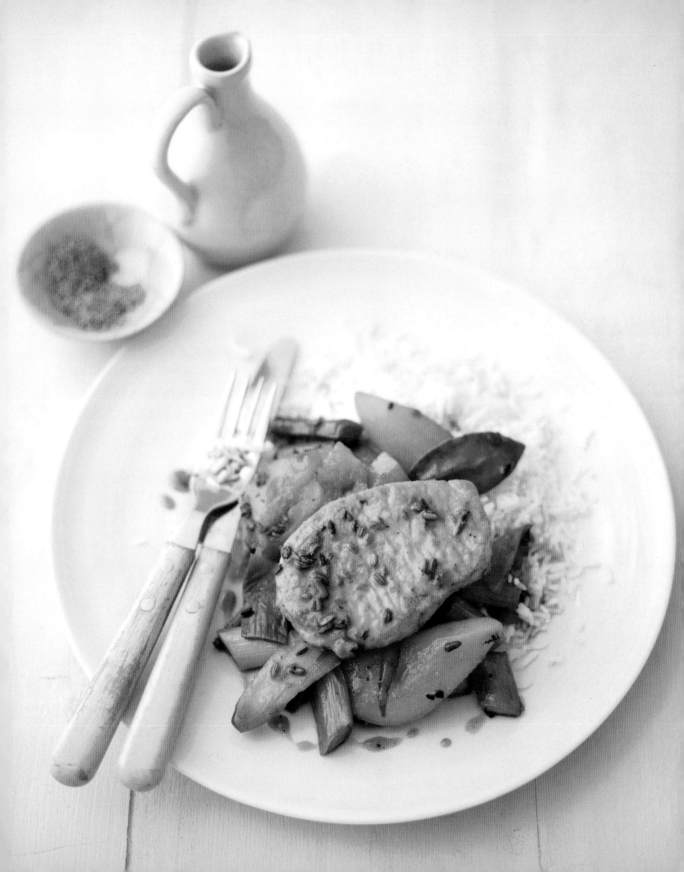

low-fat beef stroganoff

Made without the usual full-fat cream, this delicious stroganoff makes a good balanced meal served with brown rice and green veggies. And it's super quick and super easy to make, too.

serves 4

700g (1½lb) fillet steak
  (beef tenderloin), trimmed
3 tbsp plain (all-purpose)
  flour
freshly ground black pepper
1 tbsp paprika, plus extra
  for sprinkling
3 tbsp olive oil
1 onion, peeled and
  thinly sliced
225g (8oz) chestnut (cremini)
  mushrooms, sliced
1 garlic clove, peeled
  and crushed
300ml (10fl oz/1¼ cups)
  low-fat crème fraîche
1 tbsp French mustard
juice of ½ lemon, to taste

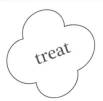
treat

1 Thinly slice the steak into 5cm (2in) strips. In a large bowl, mix the flour, some freshly ground black pepper to taste and the paprika, then coat the beef strips in the seasoned flour. Set aside.

2 Heat 2 tablespoons of the olive oil in a large deep lidded frying pan (skillet) set over a medium heat. Add the onion and fry for 5 minutes until the onion starts to soften. Add the mushrooms and garlic and fry for a few minutes or until just soft. Remove the onion and mushrooms and set aside.

3 Increase the heat and, when the pan (skillet) is hot, add the remaining olive oil, put in the beef strips and fry briskly stirring, for 3–4 minutes.

4 Return the onion and mushrooms to the pan (skillet) and season to taste with black pepper. Shake the pan (skillet) over the heat for 1 minute.

5 Reduce the heat to low and stir in the crème fraîche and mustard and cook gently for 1 minute; do not allow the liquid to boil at this point.

6 Add lemon juice to taste and serve immediately on a bed of brown rice.

lamb koftas

My in-laws make us koftas when we visit and my mother-in-law always says they are made with love. Although my mother-in-law's koftas are delicious, this is a version that is based on her recipe, but grilled (broiled) instead of deep-fried.

makes 16

for the koftas

2 white potatoes, peeled

450g (1lb) minced (ground) lamb

8 sprigs of fresh coriander (cilantro), finely chopped

8 sprigs of fresh parsley, finely chopped

1 tbsp ground cumin

1 tsp ground nutmeg

1 tsp ground cinnamon

1 garlic clove, peeled and crushed

freshly ground black pepper

2 tbsp olive oil

lemon wedges, to serve

for the dip

125g (4½oz) cucumber, deseeded and diced

275g (10oz/1¼ cups) plain yogurt

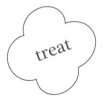
treat

1 First, preheat the grill (broiler) to its highest setting.

2 If you're using bamboo skewers, put 16 of them in hot water and leave to soak.

3 Finely grate the peeled potatoes (a good workout for your arms!) and then place in a sieve and press down for a few minutes to extract as much juice as you can – the potato gratings need to be as dry as possible.

4 Now put the minced (ground) lamb, grated potato, coriander (cilantro), parsley, cumin, nutmeg, cinnamon, garlic and freshly ground black pepper in a large bowl and mix together really well using your hands. With wet hands, roll 2 tablespoons of the mixture into an even sausage shape, then repeat with the remaining mixture to make a total of 16 koftas. Carefully skewer each kofta with a soaked wooden skewer.

5 Place the koftas on a grill (broiler) rack in the grill (broiler) pan and brush each one with a little olive oil.

6 Grill (broil) the koftas, turning frequently, for 8–10 minutes.

7 Meanwhile, mix the cucumber and yogurt together in a side dish.

8 Serve the koftas with the cucumber and yogurt dip, a green salad and lemon wedges.

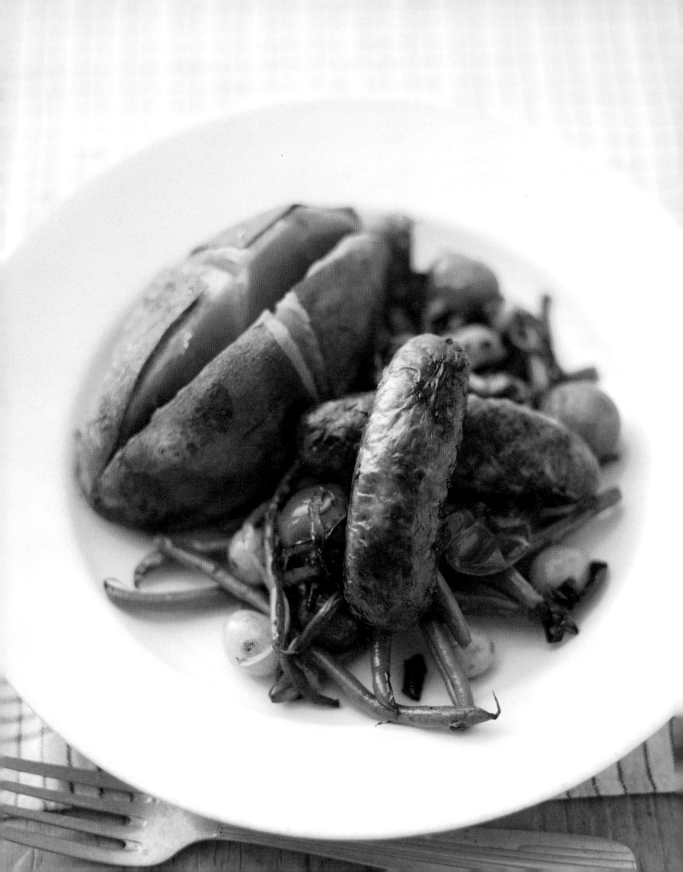

caramelised veggies with sausages and baked sweet potato

Buy only the best-quality sausages you can find, which have at least a 90 per cent meat content and that are low in salt. This dish combines the best flavours, all caramelised together. Delicious!

serves 4

4 large sweet potatoes

450g (1lb) pork sausages

1 tbsp olive oil

2 onions, peeled and sliced

1 garlic clove, peeled and
   sliced

1 tsp fennel seeds

100g (3½oz) fine green
   beans, trimmed

100g (3½oz) cherry
   tomatoes

100g (3½oz) grapes

2 tbsp apple cider vinegar

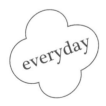
everyday

Tip:
Cooking the sausages on a grill rack prevents them from sitting in and soaking up any fat.

1 Preheat the oven to 200°C/400°F/Gas mark 6.

2 Wash the unpeeled sweet potatoes and pat them dry. Arrange them on a baking tray and pierce each one several times with a fork.

3 At the same time, prick all the sausages several times with a fork and arrange them on a wire rack set over a baking tray. Pop them in the oven with the sweet potatoes for 30–45 minutes until tender.

4 Meanwhile, heat the olive oil in a large frying pan set over a medium heat. Add the onions and cook, stirring occasionally, for about 6 minutes until starting to brown.

5 Add the garlic, fennel seeds, green beans, tomatoes and grapes and cook for another 6–8 minutes, stirring often, until the grapes and tomatoes are starting to soften and caramelise. Pour over the vinegar and swirl it around the pan. Turn off the heat and wait for the sausages to finish cooking.

6 Finally, when the sausages and sweet potatoes are done, transfer the sausages to the onion-and-grape mixture, stir and put over a medium heat for 2–3 minutes until everything is all sticky and delicious.

7 Then, place a baked sweet potato on to each plate and cut it open. To serve, pile the sausage mixture next to the sweet potato.

sticky pork steaks with pearl barley salad

This is a family favourite – the sticky pork steaks are a great hit with the children and they'll happily have a go at the salad, too.

serves 4

4 lean pork steaks, each weighing about 150g (5oz)

2 tbsp tomato purée (paste)

1 tbsp clear honey

1 tsp fennel seeds

1 garlic clove, peeled and crushed

2 tsp Worcestershire sauce

zest and juice of 1 orange

200g (7oz/1 cup) pearl barley

seeds of 1 pomegranate

4 spring onions (scallions), trimmed and sliced

2 tbsp chopped fresh mint

200g (7oz) cherry tomatoes, halved

1 tbsp olive oil

lemon wedges, to serve

1 Place the pork steaks in an ovenproof dish. Mix the tomato purée, honey, fennel seeds, garlic, Worcestershire sauce and orange zest together and pour the mixture over the steaks. Turn the steaks to coat in the sauce, then cover and leave in the refrigerator to marinate for at least 30 minutes.

2 Preheat the oven to 220ºC/425ºF/Gas mark 7.

3 When ready to cook, place the pork in the oven and cook for 20–25 minutes until the meat is cooked and the sauce is sticky.

4 Meanwhile, cook the pearl barley according to the packet instructions, then drain. Allow it to cool a little but, while it is still warm, toss through the pomegranate seeds, spring onions (scallions), mint, cherry tomatoes, orange juice and olive oil.

5 Serve the sticky pork beside the warm pearl barley salad with lemon wedges on the side.

everyday

aromatic beef casserole

I love one-pot dishes that can feed a houseful. This dish has a Thai twist with the lemongrass and can be served with rice and any number of vegetables.

serves 4–6

1.5kg (3lb 4oz) stewing beef

1 stick of lemongrass

4 tbsp olive oil

2 medium onions, peeled and chopped

5 garlic cloves, peeled and crushed

12 shallots, peeled

1 litre (1¾ pints/4 cups) hot beef stock

6 tbsp shop-bought yellow bean sauce

1 tsp chilli powder

5 whole star anise

2.5cm (1in) cinnamon stick

½ tsp whole black peppercorns

2 tbsp sugar

200g (7oz) fine green beans, trimmed

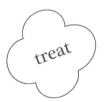
treat

1 Cut all the visible fat off the beef, then cut the meat into 2.5cm (1in) cubes. Set aside.

2 Prepare the lemongrass by cutting off the straw-like top. Cut it into 4cm (1½in) chunks and soften it by hitting it lightly with a mallet or any heavy object. Set aside.

3 Heat 2 tablespoons of the olive oil in a large, wide and lidded saucepan and, in batches, fry the meat cubes, turning to brown them all over. When nicely browned, take the meat out and set aside.

4 Reduce the heat to medium, add the remaining 2 tablespoons of olive oil to the pan and add the onions, garlic and shallots. Stir-fry for 2 minutes. Add the lemongrass and continue to stir-fry until the onions are lightly browned.

5 Return the browned meat to the pan and add the beef stock, the yellow bean sauce, chilli powder, star anise, cinnamon, whole peppercorns and sugar. Bring to the boil, then cover, reduce the heat and simmer gently for 1¼ hours, stirring every now and then.

6 Finally, take the lid off and let the sauce bubble away and reduce to a nice consistency. About 8 minutes before you are ready to serve, add the fine green beans, stir them in and let them cook in the sauce.

7 Serve with basmati rice.

Tip:
Use the best-quality stewing beef that you can find for this recipe.

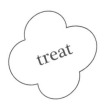
treat

stir-fried lamb with peppers

Despite the fact that this is a treat dish, it still ticks the healthy boxes, as it contains plenty of different coloured vegetables that are cooked quickly to preserve their vitamins. As with all red meat dishes, this dish should be eaten no more than once a week.

serves 2

350g (12oz) lamb neck fillet, cut into thin strips (you can ask your butcher to do this for you)

2.5cm (1in) fresh ginger, peeled and grated

1 garlic clove, peeled and crushed

4 spring onions (scallions), chopped

4 tbsp shop-bought black bean sauce

1 tbsp olive oil

1 red onion, peeled and cut into thin wedges

1 red (bell) pepper, deseeded and thinly sliced

1 green (bell) pepper, deseeded and thinly sliced

6 small florets tenderstem broccoli

1 tbsp sesame seeds

1 Prepare the lamb by trimming away any visible signs of fat. Alternatively, ask your butcher to do this for you when he cuts the lamb into strips.

2 Now, in a deep bowl, mix the lamb strips with the ginger, garlic, spring onions (scallions) and black bean sauce. Leave to marinate in the refrigerator for 30 minutes.

3 Heat the olive oil in a wok or large non-stick frying pan set over a medium heat. Add the lamb, marinade ingredients and the onion wedges and stir-fry for 5 minutes until the meat is sealed and starting to brown.

4 Add the sliced (bell) peppers and broccoli. Fry for another 5 minutes, stirring the ingredients often until the lamb is tender and the vegetables just cooked.

5 Serve sprinkled with sesame seeds, with noodles or rice.

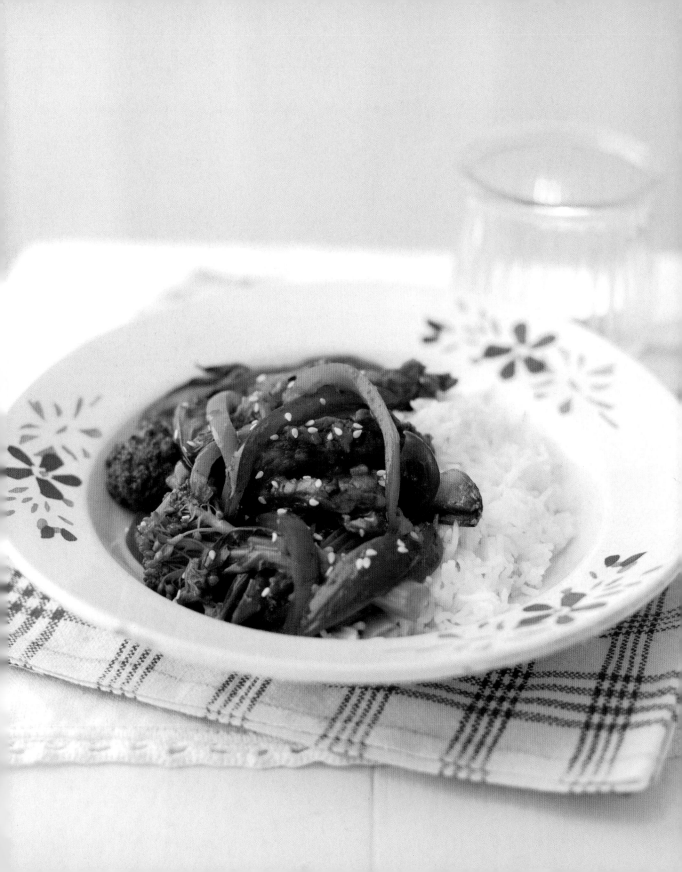

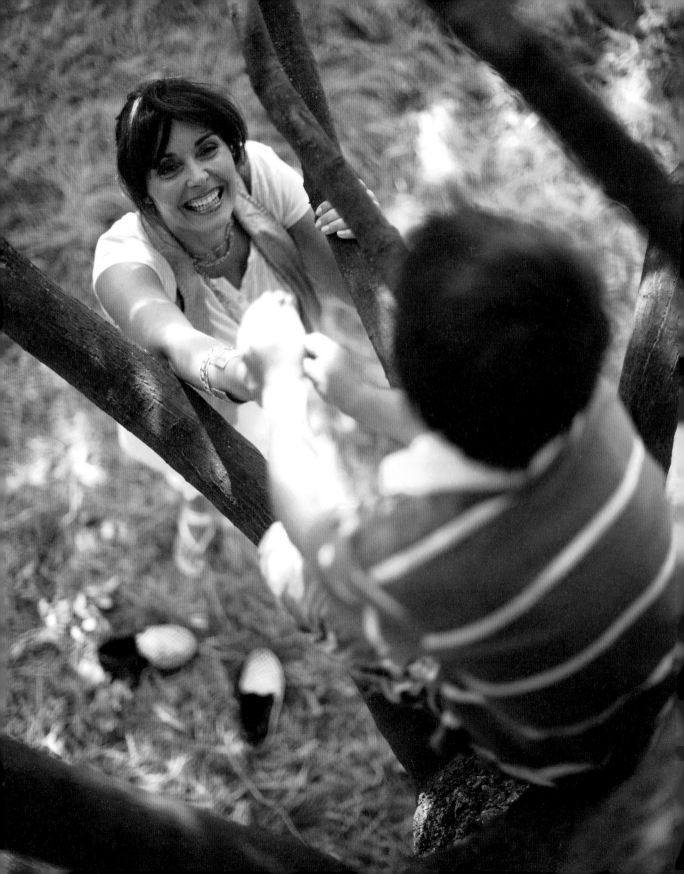

family beef hotpot

As long as you have enough time for this to cook, the preparation is quick, and then you can pop it in the oven and forget about it while you get on with something else. We often put this on for our tea, then go out for a walk with the dog to build up our appetites. As soon as we walk back in through the door, we can smell the lovely aroma of the hotpot cooking away.

serves 4–6

500g (1lb 2oz) sirloin
  beef steak

2 tbsp olive oil

2 leeks, sliced

3 celery sticks, trimmed
  and sliced

2 medium carrots, sliced

1 medium turnip, chopped

850ml (just under 1½
  pints/3½ cups) hot
  beef stock

175g (6oz) button (white)
  mushrooms, sliced

1 handful of fresh parsley,
  chopped

3 sprigs of thyme, leaves
  picked, or 1 tsp dried thyme

freshly ground black pepper

500g (1lb 2oz) white
  potatoes, peeled and sliced

1 large onion, peeled
  and sliced

1 Preheat the oven to 190°C/375°F/Gas mark 5.

2 Cut any visible fat off the steaks and cut the meat into chunks.

3 Set a large lidded ovenproof casserole dish over a high heat and add the olive oil. Add the meat a handful at a time, so that it seals and browns. Add the leeks, celery, carrots and turnip and cook, stirring from time to time, for 3–4 minutes, until slightly softened.

4 Add the hot stock, mushrooms, parsley and thyme. Season with freshly ground black pepper. Bring to the boil, then cover and transfer to the oven. Cook for 1 hour.

5 Meanwhile, parboil the potatoes for 10 minutes. Allow to cool, then slice.

6 Remove the casserole from the oven and layer the potato and onion slices over the top in overlapping layers. Return to the oven and bake, uncovered, for 45–50 minutes, until the potatoes are browned and crisp.

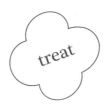

treat

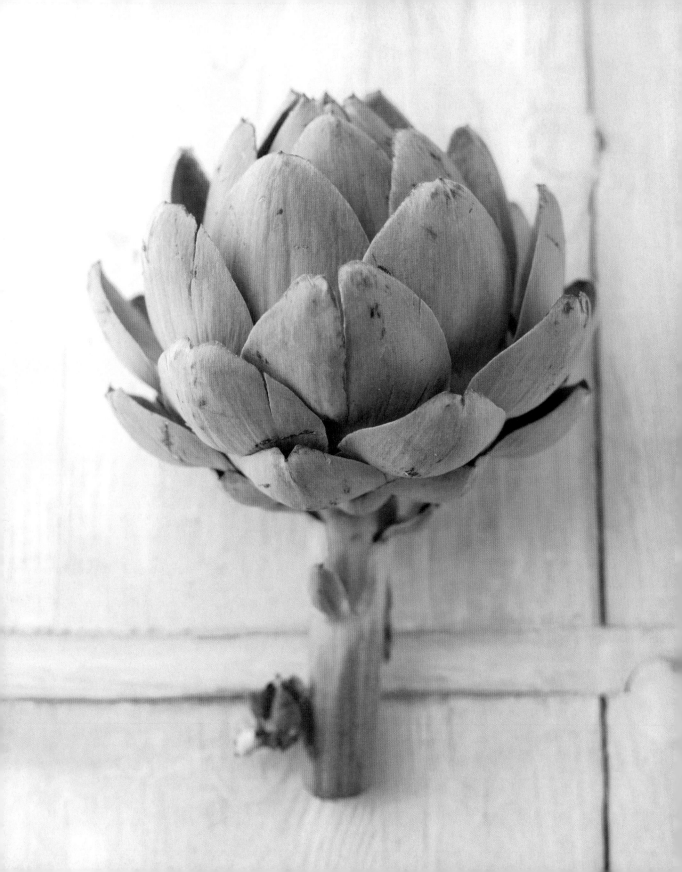

vegetarian

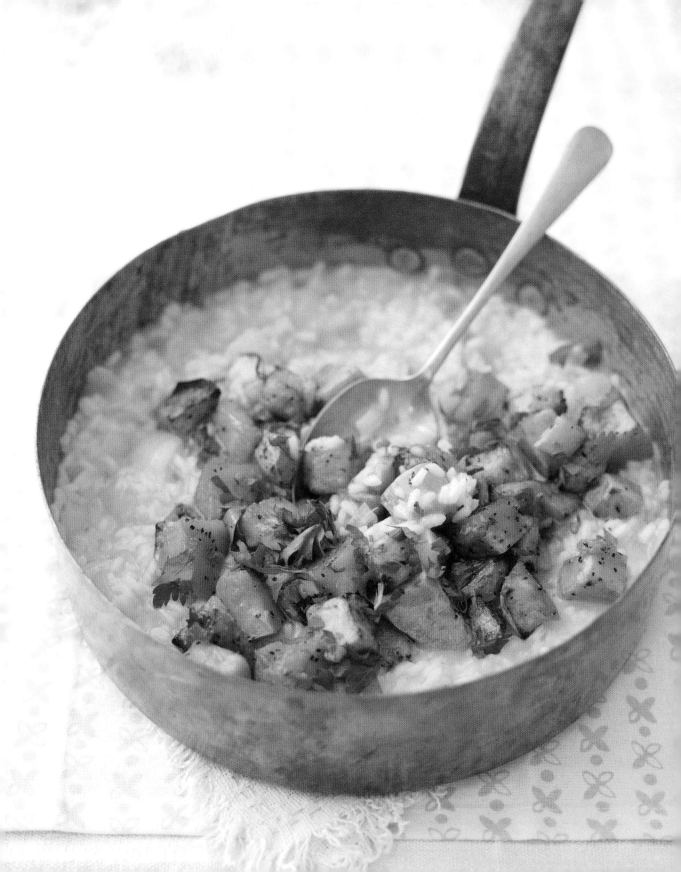

honey-roast squash risotto

Pumpkin and butternut squash are among my favourite vegetables. I find they are easy to feed to children because of their sweet flavour and gentle texture. You might guess by the yellow and orange flesh that butternut squash is packed with betacarotene and vitamin A, both of which are proven to protect us against cancer and help the heart stay healthy too. This dish is delicious, warming and low in fat.

serves 4

900g (2lb) butternut squash

3 tbsp olive oil

freshly ground black pepper

1 tsp runny honey

1 onion, peeled and roughly chopped

2 celery sticks, cut into 1cm (½in) cubes

2.5cm (1in) fresh ginger, peeled and finely grated

225g (8oz/1 cup) risotto rice

150ml (5fl oz/⅔ cup) white wine

900ml (1½ pints/3½ cups) boiling vegetable stock

juice of ½ lemon

1 small bunch of fresh flat-leaf parsley, chopped

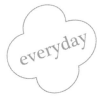

1 Preheat the oven to 220°C/425°F/Gas mark 7.

2 Peel the squash using a sharp potato peeler, cut it in half lengthways and scoop out and discard the seeds. Cut the squash flesh into 1cm (½in) cubes. Put into a large roasting tray, ensuring they are sitting in a single layer.

3 Pour over 2 tablespoons of the olive oil, season with freshly ground black pepper and toss, so that all the squash is covered with oil. Roast for about 15 minutes.

4 Remove the squash from the oven and pour over the honey, give it a good stir and return the roasting tray to the oven for a further 15 minutes or until the squash is golden brown and crisp at the edges.

5 Meanwhile, make the risotto. In a large non-stick lidded frying pan (skillet), heat the remaining tablespoon of olive oil over a high heat. Add the onion, celery and ginger and fry for a couple of minutes, then reduce the heat, cover and sauté gently for about 10 minutes. Remove the lid and add the rice and white wine. Stirring continuously, gradually add the boiling stock. Cover and cook until nearly all the liquid has been absorbed by the rice, stirring occasionally.

6 After about 20 minutes, when the rice is cooked, add the roasted squash and lemon juice and season to taste. Sprinkle in the chopped parsley and serve immediately.

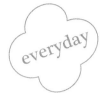

vegetable brochettes

I have marked this recipe as an everyday dish, but do ensure you use low-fat mozzarella. The veggie brochettes are easy to make, look impressive and taste divine. Whoever said vegetables are boring?

serves 6

24 large button (white) mushrooms

3 red (bell) peppers, cut into quarters

3 courgettes (zucchini), scored along the length with a fork and cut into 2cm (¾in) pieces

1 large aubergine (eggplant)

175g (6oz) half-fat mozzarella cheese, cut into 3cm x 1cm (1¼in x ½in) pieces

2 tbsp olive oil, plus extra for oiling

dash of Tabasco sauce

juice of 1 lime

a good sprinkling of chopped fresh parsley

1 tbsp finely chopped pistachio nuts or almonds

for the marinade

1 tbsp ground cumin

1 tbsp paprika

2 tbsp apple cider vinegar

2 tbsp olive oil

2 garlic cloves, peeled and crushed

dash of Tabasco sauce

1 Soak 12 wooden satay sticks that are roughly 15cm (6in) long in cold water to prevent them from burning under the grill (broiler) later.

2 Preheat the grill (broiler) to medium.

3 Combine all the marinade ingredients in a large shallow dish. Add 3 tablespoons of water and mix well. Put in the mushrooms, (bell) pepper pieces and courgette (zucchini) pieces and marinade for at least an hour.

4 Meanwhile, cut the aubergine (eggplant) into about 12 slices and cook them under the grill for 3–4 minutes until golden brown, turning once to brown evenly. Then remove from the grill and increase the grill temperature to high.

5 Lay the pieces of low-fat mozzarella on a lightly oiled baking sheet and wrap a grilled (broiled) aubergine (eggplant) slice around each of them.

6 Next, skewer the marinated vegetables on to the satay sticks, beginning and ending with a mushroom.

7 Now put the brochettes on a baking sheet and place under the hot grill (broiler) for a few minutes, turning to ensure they are well grilled (broiled) on all sides. Remove from the heat.

8 Mix the olive oil, Tabasco, lime juice and parsley in a jug (pitcher) and drizzle this over the vegetables. Finally, sprinkle with the finely chopped pistachios and serve at once.

broccoli and leek bake

This dish is so quick and easy and goes beautifully with any chicken or fish dish. It is marked as everyday because it contains only a tiny amount of cheese, which is divided between 4 portions, so well within the healthy range.

serves 4

2 tbsp olive oil

1 large onion, peeled and
   cut into wedges

2 garlic cloves, peeled and
   crushed

1 aubergine (eggplant),
   chopped

2 leeks, trimmed and cut
   into chunks

1 head of broccoli, cut into
   florets and stalks chopped

3 large flat mushrooms,
   chopped

3 sprigs of fresh rosemary,
   leaves picked and chopped

2 x 400g (14oz) tins chopped
   tomatoes

300ml (10fl oz/1¼ cups)
   vegetable stock

freshly ground black pepper

50g (2oz/⅓ cup)
   half-fat mature Cheddar
   cheese, grated

50g (2oz) pine nuts

1 Preheat the oven to 200°C/400°F/Gas mark 6.

2 Heat the olive oil in a large ovenproof casserole dish. Add the onion, garlic, aubergine (eggplant) and leeks and cook for 10–12 minutes until golden and softened.

3 Next, add the broccoli and mushrooms, half the rosemary, the tinned tomatoes and the stock. Season with freshly ground black pepper and stir well, then cover and bake in the oven for 30 minutes.

4 Meanwhile, put the grated cheese in a bowl, add the remaining rosemary and the pine nuts and season with freshly ground pepper. Set aside.

5 When the vegetables are cooked, remove from the oven, uncover and sprinkle the cheese and pine nut mixture over. Return to the oven and cook, uncovered, for 5–10 minutes until the top is nicely golden.

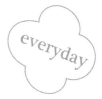
everyday

gift-wrapped baked vegetables

Opening this lovely parcel of colourful wholesome, healthy and sweet-tasting veggies is almost as good as eating it. I've listed my favourite vegetables here, but if you want to make swaps for your favourites, just go ahead. Treat the weights of vegetables as approximate – obviously, if you have a little spare of something, use it!

serves 4

115g (4oz) carrots

115g (4oz) celeriac
  (celery root)

115g (4oz) raw
  beetroot (beet)

115g (4oz) sweet potatoes

115g (4oz) parsnips

115g (4oz) shallots, peeled

115g (4oz) new potatoes

8 garlic cloves, unpeeled

3 tbsp olive oil

1 tbsp white wine

1 tsp celery salt

freshly ground black pepper

handful of fresh
  rosemary sprigs

handful of chopped
  fresh parsley

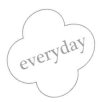

1 Preheat the oven to 190°C/375°F/Gas mark 5.

2 Prepare 4 sheets of baking parchment, cutting each one to 20cm x 20cm (8in x 8in). Set aside.

3 Wash all the veggies and cut everything (except the shallots and new potatoes) up into 3cm (1¼in) chunks.

4 Mix the cut vegetables, potatoes, whole shallots and unpeeled garlic with the olive oil, white wine, celery salt and freshly ground black pepper.

5 Divide the vegetables equally between the sheets of baking parchment and wrap the parchment around the veggies, folding the edges tightly together to form a bag. Before folding over the last edge to close the parcels, throw in some rosemary sprigs and chopped parsley. Then place the parcels closely together on a baking tray. Pop the tray into the oven for 35–40 minutes.

6 Serve the vegetables in their wrappers straight from the oven.

Tip:
In this recipe I use 1 teaspoon of celery salt, which is fine when divided between the 4 parcels. It really helps to bring out the flavour of the vegetables.

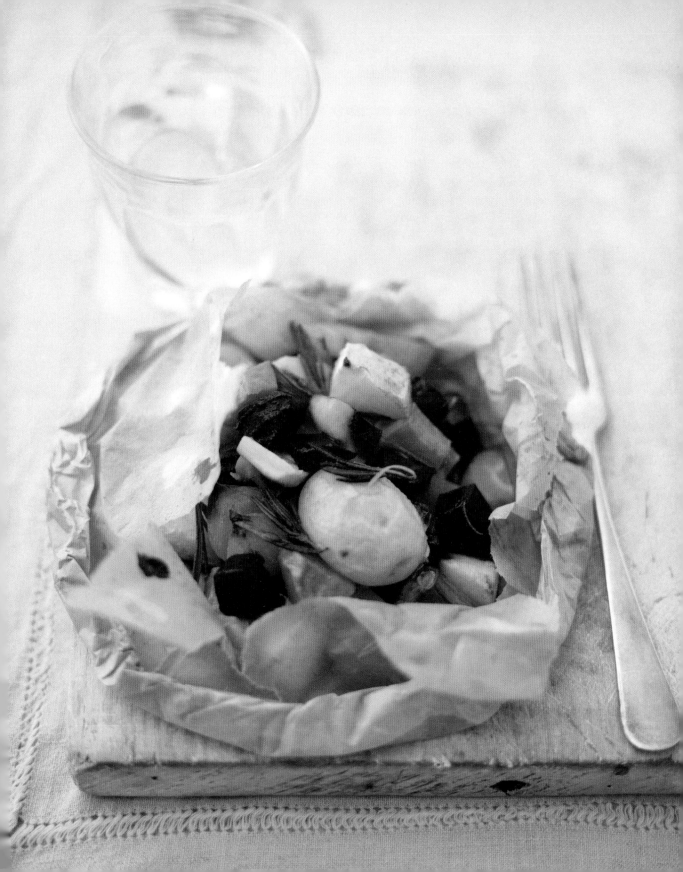

green bean and mangetout stir-fry

A delicious way to eat your greens! I like to have this on its own but, of course, you can serve it as a side dish or starter. Although it contains some soy sauce, which does contain salt, I have still listed it as an everyday dish because of the great 'green' content. It's OK to use a little salt in cooking as long as you don't have too much in any processed food. If you feel that your salt content needs attention, miss out the soy sauce and substitute lemon juice.

serves 4

2 tbsp light soy sauce or lemon juice

2 tsp clear honey

2 tbsp olive oil

2 spring onions (scallions), trimmed and sliced

225g (8oz) fine green beans

225g (8oz) mangetout (snow peas) or sugar snap peas

½ green (bell) pepper, deseeded and sliced

2 red chillies, deseeded and sliced

½ tsp ground star anise

1 garlic clove, peeled and crushed

1 Mix the soy sauce or lemon juice and honey together in a small bowl and set aside.

2 Heat the olive oil in a non-stick wok or heavy-based frying pan (skillet) set over a high heat. When the oil is almost smoking, reduce the heat to medium and throw in the spring onions (scallions) and all the green vegetables and stir-fry for 3 minutes.

3 Next, add the red chillies, the star anise and the garlic and stir-fry for a further 30 seconds. Add the soy/honey sauce to the wok and cook for 2 minutes, tossing constantly to ensure all the veggies are covered in the delicious sauce.

4 Pop the stir-fry into a warmed serving dish and serve immediately.

wholewheat penne pasta with tomato chilli sauce

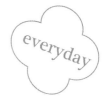

everyday

Many shop-bought pasta sauces have really high salt and sugar contents, so home-made is better. This sauce is easy to make and absolutely full of flavour, but without any of the unhealthy ingredients found in processed pasta sauces. The red wine and tomatoes and garlic all have great antioxidant properties and, if you use wholewheat pasta, you have good fibre, too.

serves 6

2 tbsp olive oil

1 large onion, peeled and finely chopped

2 garlic cloves, peeled and crushed

2 red chillies, deseeded and finely chopped

200ml (7fl oz/¾ cup) red wine

1 kg (2lb 2oz) ripe plum tomatoes, chopped

freshly ground black pepper

500g (1lb 2oz) dried wholewheat penne pasta

10 fresh basil leaves, torn, plus extra for sprinkling

1 Heat the olive oil in a large pan set over a low heat. Add the onion and cook for about 10 minutes until soft.

2 Now add the garlic and chillies to the pan and cook for 2 minutes. Pour in the wine, bring to the boil and allow it to bubble for 1–2 minutes.

3 Add the tomatoes and bring to the boil, then reduce the heat to low and simmer, stirring occasionally, until the tomatoes have reduced to a thick sauce. This will take about 50 minutes. Season with freshly ground black pepper to taste.

4 About 10 minutes before the sauce is ready, cook the pasta according to the packet instructions.

5 Drain the pasta well, adding a little of the cooking water to the tomato sauce to thin it. Return the pasta to the pan and add the tomato sauce and torn basil. Toss the mixture and serve scattered with a few extra basil leaves.

Tip:
Feel free to add cooked chicken or canned tuna to this pasta dish to bulk it out a bit.

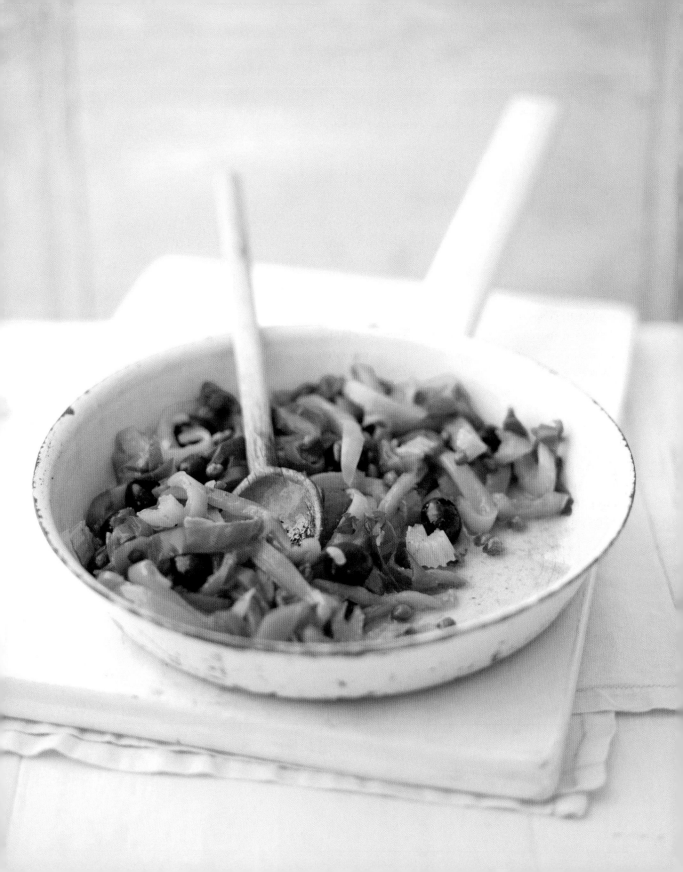

french pepper stew

It always amazes me how people think that eating a healthy diet in some way is depriving them of tasty food. This simple stew should be called 'vitamin bomb in a bowl'. I'm addicted to it!

serves 6–8 as a side dish

2 garlic cloves, peeled and crushed

3 tbsp olive oil

3 red (bell) peppers, deseeded and sliced

3 orange (bell) peppers, deseeded and sliced

2 green (bell) peppers, deseeded and sliced

2 celery sticks, sliced

freshly ground black pepper

2 tbsp capers in brine, rinsed

18 black olives pitted

1 tbsp chopped fresh flat-leaf parsley

1 Fry the garlic in the olive oil in a large pan set over a medium heat for 1 minute. Add the sliced (bell) peppers and celery and season with freshly ground black pepper.

2 Cover the pan and cook over a low heat for 40 minutes, stirring regularly.

3 Finally, add the capers, olives and parsley and stir. Serve immediately while hot, or put the stew in the refrigerator and serve it cold later.

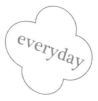
everyday

pumpkin and mushroom lasagne

Whether or not you are a vegetarian, this dish is gorgeous to eat and as easy as pie to make. And it's so good for you – pumpkins are packed with vitamins. Serve this lasagne with some wholemeal bread and a salad or some green veggies.

serves 6

approximately 1.5kg
 (3lb 4oz) pumpkin

2 tbsp olive oil

4 garlic cloves, peeled
 and crushed

750g (1lb 10oz) mushrooms,
 (button/white and
 shiitake), thinly sliced

freshly ground black pepper

350ml (12fl oz/1½ cups) milk

4 shallots, peeled and
 thinly sliced

1 handful of chopped fresh
 sage (or 2 tsp dried sage)

250g (9oz) lasagne
 verde sheets

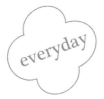

1 Preheat the oven to 200°C/400°F/Gas mark 6.

2 Cut the pumpkin in half lengthways. Peel and deseed half of the pumpkin and cut it into 2cm (¾in) cubes. Set aside. Remove the seeds from the remaining pumpkin half, but do not peel it.

3 Lightly coat the bottom of a baking tray with a little olive oil and place the unpeeled half of the pumpkin on the baking tray, cut-side down. Roast it for 35–40 minutes or until very soft. Remove from the oven and set aside to cool.

4 Meanwhile, put the remaining olive oil in a large frying pan set over a medium heat. Add half of the garlic, the cubed pumpkin and the mushrooms and cook for 8–10 minutes or until tender. Season with freshly ground black pepper. Remove from the heat and leave to cool.

5 Now, in a medium-sized saucepan, combine the milk, shallots, remaining garlic and the sage and cook over a medium heat, bringing the milk to the boil. Cover, remove from the heat and set aside.

6 Scrape the flesh from the roasted pumpkin half. Place it in a large bowl and mash with a potato masher. Add the milk mixture and mash to combine. Season to taste with freshly ground black pepper.

7 Take a 24cm x 24cm (9in x 9in) square casserole dish and smear a tiny bit of olive oil on the bottom to

stop everything from sticking. Then put the lasagne together in layers, alternating the mushroom and pumpkin mixture, the pasta sheets and the pumpkin mash. Ensure you finish with a layer of pumpkin mash on top.

8 Cover the casserole dish with foil and bake in the oven for 30 minutes. Remove the foil and bake for a further 10 minutes.

baked red peppers

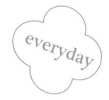
everyday

Serve this up as a side dish or light lunch. The preparation takes only minutes, then the dish cooks away in the oven, allowing you to get on with something much more fun! I like to use red (bell) peppers, but you can use any colour you like.

serves 4

4 red (bell) peppers

1 large onion, peeled and
   cut into wedges

2 medium tomatoes,
   finely diced

1 medium fennel bulb,
   trimmed and cut
   into wedges

3 garlic cloves, peeled
   and crushed

drizzle of olive oil

freshly ground black pepper

200g (7oz) low-fat
   mozzarella cheese, sliced

1 Preheat the oven to 130°C/250°F/Gas mark ½.

2 Cut the (bell) peppers in half lengthways and remove the core. Put them in a suitably sized baking tray (cookie sheet).

3 Put the onion, diced tomatoes, fennel and garlic in a bowl, drizzle over some olive oil and season with black pepper. Give it all a good stir to coat all the vegetables with the oil.

4 Stuff the (bell) peppers with the vegetable mixture and bake in the oven for 1 hour and 20 minutes.

5 Finally, take the (bell) peppers out of the oven and place the slices of low-fat mozzarella over the tops of the (bell) peppers. You can either grill (broil) them for 2–3 minutes until the cheese starts to bubble, or increase the oven temperature to 200°C/400°F/Gas mark 6 and put them back in the oven for an extra 5 minutes.

chilli beans on toast

Beans and pulses contain as much protein as fillet steak, but at a fraction of the cost. And they have many more health benefits – they are high in fibre, folate, potassium and zinc.

serves 4

2 x 400g (14oz) tins mixed
  beans, drained and rinsed
1 red chilli, deseeded and
  chopped (or 1 tsp chilli
  flakes/red pepper flakes)
1 garlic clove, peeled
  and crushed
500g (1lb 2oz) carton of
  passata (strained tomatoes)
2 tsp light muscovado
  (brown) sugar
2 tbsp balsamic vinegar
4 slices wholemeal
  (wholewheat)
  bread, toasted

1 Put all the ingredients (except for the bread – obviously!) in a medium-sized saucepan set over a medium heat and cook until starting to bubble. Reduce the heat slightly and simmer for 4–5 minutes.

2 Meanwhile, toast the bread – no need for butter!

3 Serve the beans on top of the toast, piping hot.

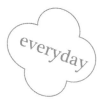
everyday

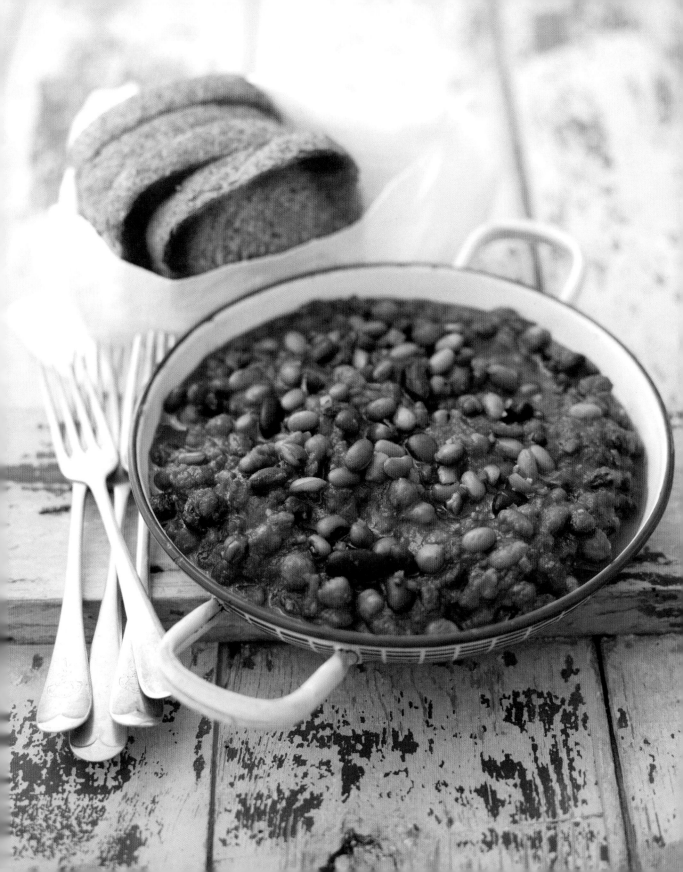

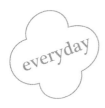

stuffed roast butternut squash

The two ways of cooking the squash in this dish enhance the intensity of its delicious flavour while maintaining all of the goodness. If you like butternut squash, you'll love this!

serves 4 as a side dish or 2 as a main course

2 butternut squashes, each weighing approximately 500g (1lb 2oz)

1 tbsp olive oil

freshly ground black pepper

1 onion, peeled and chopped

1 garlic clove, peeled and sliced

1 red (bell) pepper, deseeded and chopped

200g (7oz) cherry tomatoes, halved

1 tsp sugar

2 tbsp balsamic vinegar

4 spring onions (scallions), trimmed and chopped

50g (2oz/⅓ cup) pine nuts

torn fresh basil leaves, to garnish

1 Preheat the oven to 180°C/350°F/Gas mark 4.

2 Cut the butternut squashes in half lengthways. Remove the seeds, brush with a little of the olive oil, then season with freshly ground black pepper. Place the halves on a baking tray cut-side up and bake for 20 minutes or until the squashes are cooked through. Carefully cut out a little of the flesh from each half, dice it and set aside.

3 Meanwhile, heat the rest of the olive oil in a large pan set over a medium heat. Cook the onion, garlic and red (bell) pepper for 5 minutes, then add the tomatoes and sugar. Reduce the heat and simmer for 10–15 minutes.

4 Next, stir in the balsamic vinegar, spring onions (scallions) and pine nuts and add the reserved diced butternut squash. Season again with freshly ground black pepper.

5 Squeeze all the mixture into the hollows of the baked squash halves and return them to the oven for an extra 10 minutes.

6 Remove from the oven, scatter with torn basil leaves and serve.

rainbow peppers and bulgur wheat

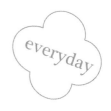
everyday

I often talk about the importance of having a rainbow of colours when it comes to your daily intake of vegetables. This dish gets top marks.

serves 4

125g (4½oz/1 cup) bulgur or cracked wheat

4 tbsp olive oil

1 large onion, peeled and thinly sliced

½ red (bell) pepper, deseeded and thinly sliced

½ green (bell) pepper, deseeded and thinly sliced

½ yellow (bell) pepper, deseeded and thinly sliced

2 tsp ground coriander

2 tsp ground cumin

100g (3½oz/1 cup) flaked (slivered) almonds

60g (2½oz/⅓ cup) raisins

freshly ground black pepper

1 Make up the bulgur or cracked wheat according to the packet instructions. You'll know it's cooked when the grains are soft.

2 Meanwhile, in a large, non-stick pan, heat the olive oil over a medium heat and add the onion. Fry for 5 minutes until starting to soften. Then add the thinly sliced peppers and sauté for another 5 minutes.

3 After this time, add the coriander and cumin and cook for 1 minute stirring continuously.

4 Now reduce the heat to low and add the almonds and raisins and cook for another couple of minutes.

5 Finally, stir in the cooked bulgur or cracked wheat and season with freshly ground black pepper. Warm through and serve.

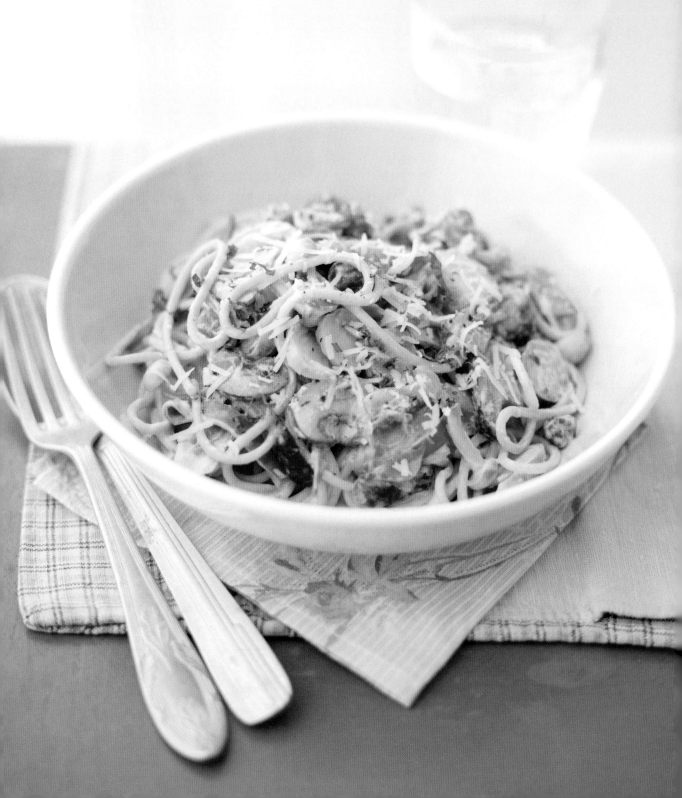

creamy spaghetti with brussels sprouts and mushrooms

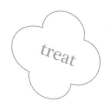
treat

Originally, I made this dish using wholewheat fettuccine, but as it is hard to find on the high street, I've adapted it to use spaghetti. But if you do find some wholewheat fettuccine, give it a try. Whichever pasta shape you use, this dish is a healthy alternative to the usual creamy pasta.

serves 4

350g (12oz) wholewheat spaghetti

1 tbsp olive oil

200g (7oz) mixed mushrooms, sliced

200g (7oz) Brussels sprouts, thinly sliced

200g (7oz) mangetout (snow peas), thinly sliced

1 garlic clove, peeled and crushed

2 tbsp sherry vinegar or red wine vinegar

4 tbsp low-fat crème fraîche

50g (2oz) low-fat mature hard cheese (Cheddar cheese), finely grated

freshly ground black pepper

chopped fresh curly parsley, to serve

1 Cook the pasta according the packet instructions. Drain, return to the pan and set aside.

2 Meanwhile, heat the olive oil in a large frying pan set over a medium heat. Add the mushrooms, Brussels sprouts and mangetout (snow peas) and cook, stirring often, for about 8 minutes, by which time the mushrooms will have released their liquid.

3 Now add the crushed garlic and cook for 1 minute.

4 Add the vinegar, scraping up any tasty bits that have stuck to the pan. Bring to the boil over a high heat, then immediately take the pan off the heat.

5 Finally, stir in the low-fat crème fraîche, most of the cheese and a good sprinkling of freshly ground black pepper. Serve straight away, with the remaining cheese on top and with the parsley sprinkled over.

Tip:
I have marked this dish as a treat simply because it contains some dairy. But don't let this put you off – it will still offer you some wonderful nutrition as well as a delicious experience!

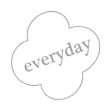

celeriac casserole in cabbage leaves

Wholesome, nutritious, seriously low in fat, and with a lovely flavour – this is a great dish to entice children to eat more greens!

serves 6

1 Savoy cabbage

50g (2oz) French (green) beans

3 tbsp olive oil

1 red onion, peeled and finely chopped

1 red (bell) pepper, deseeded and very finely diced

2 garlic cloves, peeled and crushed

3 tsp garam masala

½ tsp ground coriander

2 tsp paprika

750g (1lb 10oz) potatoes, peeled and diced

750g (1lb 10oz) celeriac (celery root), peeled, cut into 1cm (½in) thick slices, then diced

freshly ground black pepper

250g (9oz) chestnut (cremini) or button (white) mushrooms, quartered

1 tsp low-salt soy sauce

1 tsp shop-bought chilli sauce

juice of 1 lemon

good handful of fresh parsley, chopped

1 Place 225ml (8fl oz/1 cup) of water in a jug (pitcher) by your stove.

2 Separate 6 outer leaves from the cabbage and blanch them in boiling water for just 1 minute. Drain and refresh in cold water. Place them decoratively in a serving bowl and set aside.

3 Now blanch the French (green) beans in the same water for 2 minutes, then drain the beans and dice them. Set aside.

4 Halve and quarter the remaining cabbage. Cut out the core and cut a piece of it weighing about 100g (3½oz). Shred this with a long sharp knife.

5 Now, heat 2 tablespoons of the olive oil in a large saucepan set over a medium heat. Add the onion, (bell) pepper and garlic and fry for 5 minutes until soft. Add the garam masala, coriander and paprika and fry for 1–2 minutes, adding to 2–3 tablespoons of water from your jug (pitcher) to loosen the spices.

6 Next, add the potatoes and stir over the heat for 2–3 minutes. Add the celeriac, freshly ground black pepper and keep stirring over a low heat adding 2–3 tablespoons of water from your jug (pitcher) from time to time to prevent sticking.

7 Now add the mushrooms, the low-salt soy sauce and the chilli sauce and cook down for a couple of minutes. Add

in the shredded cabbage and continue to stir, adding a little water from your jug (pitcher) from time to time.

8 After 25–30 minutes, the potatoes and celeriac (celery root) should be tender but not falling apart. To serve, add the lemon juice, then the cooked French (green) beans and heat through.

9 Spoon the casserole mixture on to the blanched outer leaves of the cabbage, garnish with plenty of chopped parsley, pour over any remaining liquid from the pan and serve hot.

boulangère potatoes

Similar to a dish that uses gallons of double (heavy) cream, this low-fat version takes some time to cook in the oven, but it's definitely worth the wait. It contains only a tiny amount of butter, so I have happily marked it as an everyday dish.

serves 4

25g (1oz/2tbsp) butter

700g (1½lb) floury (mealy) potatoes, peeled and very thinly sliced

1 large onion, peeled very thinly sliced

freshly ground black pepper

200ml (7fl oz/¾ cup) vegetable stock

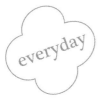

1 Preheat the oven to 170°C/325°F/Gas mark 3.

2 Grease a pie dish that is approximately 28cm x 23cm x 7.5cm deep (11in x 9in x 3in deep) with a little of the butter and arrange the potatoes and onion in layers in the dish, adding freshly ground black pepper as you go. Arrange the top layer of potatoes in overlapping slices and dot with the remaining butter.

3 Pour in the stock. Press the potatoes down firmly – they should be completely submerged in the stock.

4 Bake in the oven for 2 hours or until the potatoes are tender and the top browned.

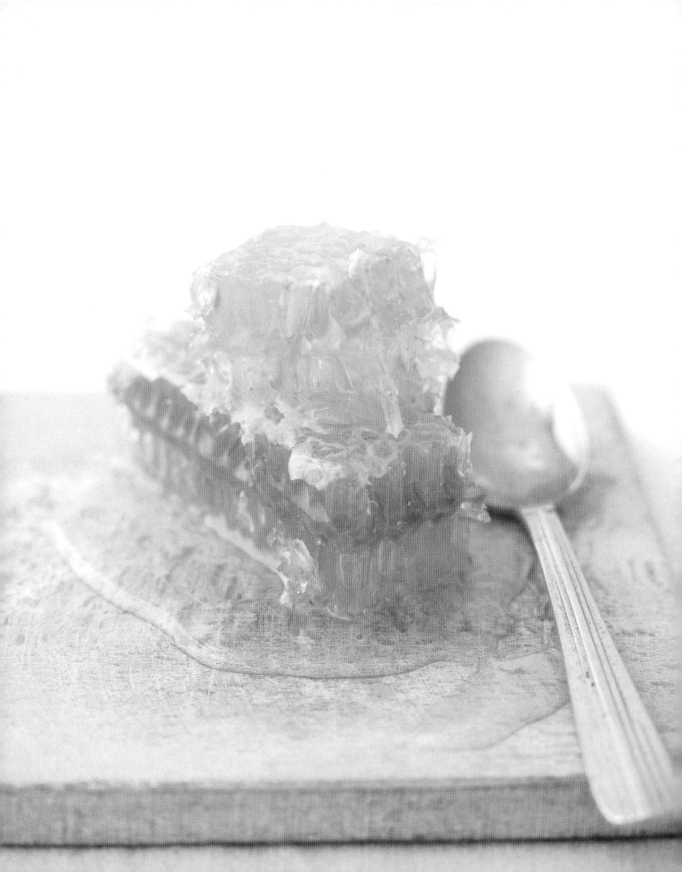

desserts

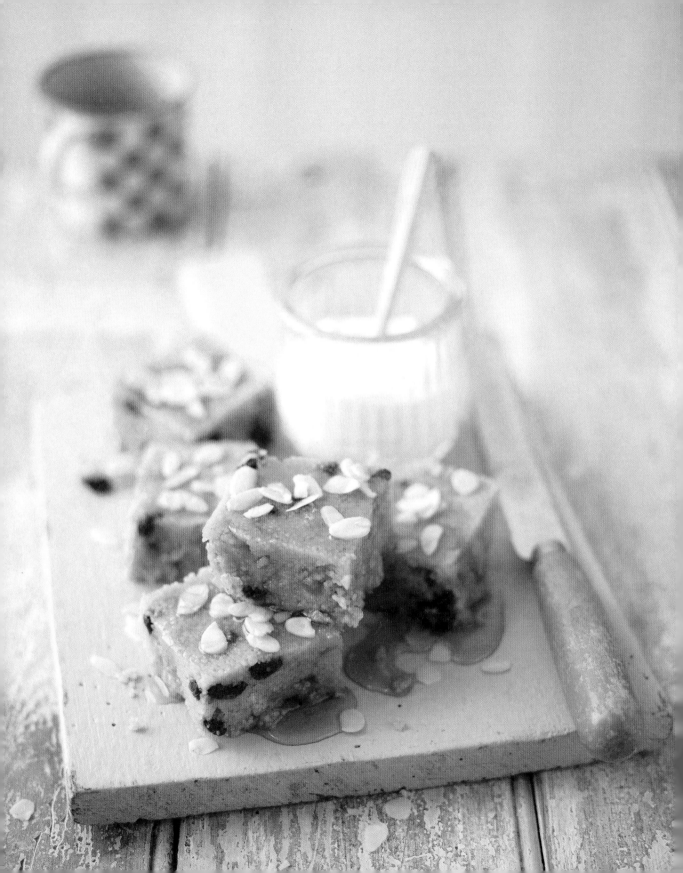

Mediterranean couscous cake

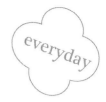
everyday

I first ate a cake like this in Cyprus and loved it, but it had been drowned in a sweet syrup that made it just a little too much. This recipe is based on that Mediterranean cake but, without too much of the sweet stuff. With no added sugar or fat, I've marked this cake as an everyday dish – enjoy!

serves 16

500g (1lb 2oz/2½ cups)
   couscous
200g (7oz/1⅛ cups) ready-
   to-eat dried apricots,
   finely chopped
200g (7oz/1½ cups) raisins
½ tsp ground cinnamon
3 tsp lime juice
3 tsp orange juice
450g (1lb) clear honey, plus
   2 tbsp extra for drizzling
2 tbsp flaked
   (slivered) almonds
low-fat Greek yogurt,
   to serve

1 Line a 23cm (9in) square loose-bottomed cake tin with baking parchment.

2 Place the couscous in a large bowl and pour in 650ml (just a little over 1 pint/2¾ cups) of boiling water and leave to stand for 10 minutes.

3 Meanwhile, put all the other ingredients, except the flaked (slivered) almonds, into a large saucepan set over a low heat and cook for about 5 minutes until the fruit is nicely softened and all the ingredients are working together.

4 Take the saucepan off the heat, add the couscous and mix together very well.

5 Put all of the mixture into the lined cake tin and press down hard using the back of a wooden spoon. Drizzle with the extra honey and sprinkle over the flaked almonds. Leave the cake (at room temperature) to set, then serve each portion with a dollop of Greek yogurt.

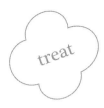
treat

sweetie sesame bananas

Bananas are healthy, filling and conveniently wrapped! This is a very easy dessert recipe with only a small amount of sugar per serving.

serves 4

4 ripe medium bananas, cut into 5cm (2in) pieces

3 tbsp lemon juice

115g (4oz/½ cup) caster (superfine) sugar

2 tbsp sesame seeds

150ml (5fl oz/⅔ cup) low-fat fromage frais

1 tsp vanilla essence (extract)

1 Put the chunks of banana in a large bowl and pour over the lemon juice immediately. This will help prevent the bananas discolouring.

2 Next, put the sugar and 2 tablespoons of cold water in a small saucepan and heat gently, stirring constantly, until the sugar dissolves. Bring to the boil and cook for 5–6 minutes or until the mixture caramelises and turns golden brown.

3 Meanwhile, drain the bananas and put on to a non-stick baking sheet, leaving a good space between each piece.

4 When the caramel is ready drizzle it over the bananas straight away before it begins to set. Then quickly sprinkle over the sesame seeds and serve with a dollop of low-fat fromage frais drizzled with a drop of vanilla essence (extract).

apricot purée and muesli pot

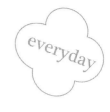

A wonderful trick for brightening up breakfast or turning muesli into a delicious (but very healthy) dessert is to combine it with this yummy apricot purée.

serves 4

350g (12oz/2 cups) soft
   dried apricots
300ml (11fl oz/1¼ cups)
   orange juice
12 tbsp your favourite sugar-
   free muesli
8 tbsp low-fat fromage frais
4 tsp crushed pistachio nuts
4 sprigs of fresh mint,
   to decorate

1 Put the apricots and orange juice in a small saucepan and bring to the boil over a medium heat. Reduce the heat, cover and simmer for 25–30 minutes or until the apricots are very tender.

2 Remove the apricot mixture from the heat, transfer to a bowl and allow to cool, then chill in the refrigerator for 30 minutes. (You can make the purée ahead of time and store it in the refrigerator for up to 5 days.)

3 Once chilled, blend the fruit either with a hand-held blender or in a liquidiser. Add a little more orange juice if it is too thick.

4 Take 4 medium wine glasses and layer up the muesli, fromage frais and apricot purée to make a strip effect. Sprinkle each glass with the crushed pistachio nuts and serve with a sprig of mint to decorate.

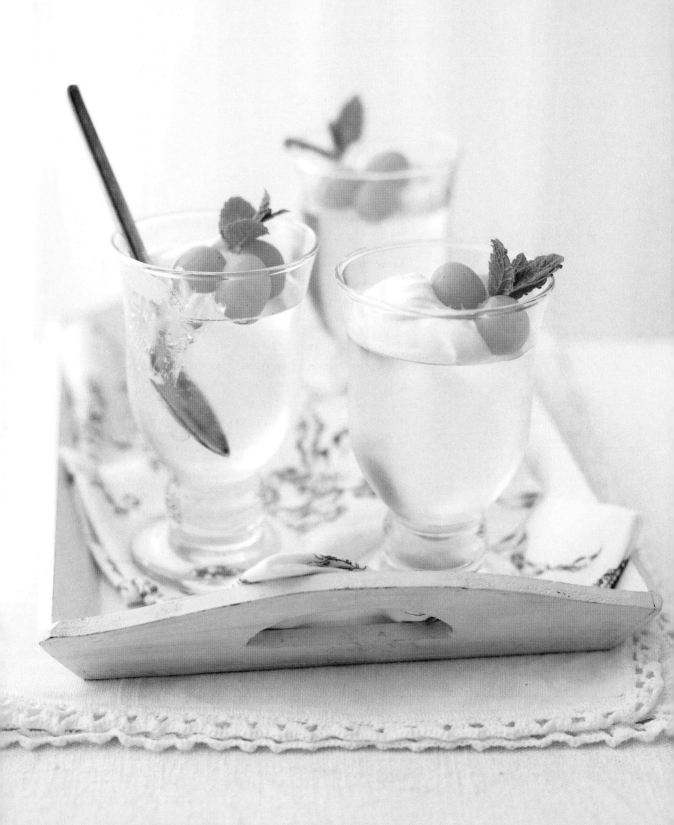

elderflower jelly

My children call this champagne jelly, but it's actually made with elderflower cordial – although I guess for a special occasion you could crack open a bottle of the real stuff! If you are serving this at a party, the jellies can be made up to two days ahead of time and stored in the refrigerator.

serves 4

600ml (1 pint/2½ cups)
  sparkling water

75ml (3fl oz/⅓ cup)
  elderflower cordial

4 gelatine (gelatin) leaves
  that are approximately
  7cm x 11cm (2¾in x 4½in)

to serve

low-fat fromage frais

1 handful of seedless
  green grapes

4 sprigs of fresh mint

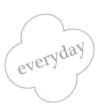
everyday

1 Pour the cold sparkling water into a jug (pitcher) and stir in the cordial.

2 Place the gelatine (gelatin) leaves in a small heatproof bowl and add 4 tablespoons of the elderflower mixture. Leave to soak for 10 minutes or until the gelatine (gelatin) is very soft.

3 Next, place the bowl with the gelatine (gelatin) leaves over a pan of barely simmering water and stir until the gelatine (gelatin) has completely dissolved. Add this dissolved gelatine mixture to the remaining elderflower mixture and stir well. Pour into 4 wine glasses, and chill in the refrigerator for 2–3 hours.

4 Serve the jelly in the glasses, topped with low-fat fromage frais, a few grapes and a sprig of fresh mint.

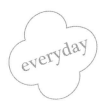

a lovely pear of plums!

There are so many wonderful ways of eating fruit. You don't need to add any extra sugar, as fruit has plenty of its own – and, when heated slowly, the flavour and sweetness becomes even more intense. This dish had a great combination of antioxidant-giving fruits that will help keep the bugs away! Serve it with low-fat fromage frais or crème fraîche.

serves 4

4 medium dessert pears, peeled, cored and sliced

6 medium plums, halved

zest and juice of 1 large orange

½ tsp ground cinnamon

225g (8oz/1½ cups) frozen blueberries or forest fruits

4 tbsp low-fat fromage frais or crème fraîche

2 tsp sunflower seeds

1 Put the pears, plums, half the orange zest, the orange juice, cinnamon and frozen berries in a large lidded saucepan with 3 tablespoons of cold water. Bring to the boil over a high heat, then reduce the heat to medium and simmer gently, with the lid on, for 10–15 minutes or until the fruit is tender. Spoon into 4 serving dishes and allow to cool slightly.

2 Mix the fromage frais or crème fraîche with the sunflower seeds and remaining orange zest and place a dollop on top of each serving.

exotic fruit meringues

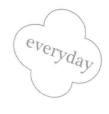

Marked as a treat because of the sugar content, this dish still offers healthy fruit and protein from the egg white. And the great news is that it's fat free!

serves 6

6 egg whites

325g (11oz/1⅝ cups) golden caster (superfine) sugar

1 tsp cornflour (cornstarch)

4 passion fruits

100ml (3½fl oz/⅓cup) mango juice

1 ripe mango, peeled and thinly sliced

1 ripe papaya, peeled, deseeded and thinly sliced

seeds of 1 pomegranate

1 Preheat the oven to 110°C/220°F/Gas mark ¼ (or its lowest setting).

2 Line a baking sheet with baking parchment.

3 Beat the egg whites until very stiff, beating either by hand or in with an electric whisk. Add the golden caster sugar a bit at a time, then gently beat in the cornflour (cornstarch).

4 Using two spoons, shape 6 large or 12 smaller meringues and place them on the prepared baking parchment.

5 Bake for about 1–1½ hours until crisp, then turn off the oven and open the door, leaving the meringues to cool in the oven.

6 Cut the passion fruits in half, scoop out the pulp and rub it through a sieve to extract the juice (reserve the seeds). Mix the passion fruit juice with the mango juice and pour into a sauté pan together with the mango and papaya slices. Add the passion fruit seeds to the pan and bring to the boil, then switch off the heat and leave to cool. Spread some of the fruit and juice over each plate, then top with either one large or two small meringues, then the rest of the fruit. Sprinkle with the pomegranate seeds to serve.

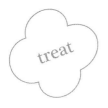
treat

apricot
and pistachio tart

This is a really easy, impressive-looking dessert. Erring on the side of caution, I've marked this dish as a treat because of the puff pastry but when served in small portions, this is still a nutritional serving because of the apricots and pistachios. So enjoy this on a special occasion, shared with friends.

serves 4

75g (3oz/½ cup) roasted pistachio nuts (shelled weight), plus a few extra for sprinkling

5 tbsp clear honey

1 tsp ground cinnamon

zest and juice of 1 orange

375g (13oz) shop-bought ready rolled puff pastry

10 apricots, halved and pitted

1 egg, beaten

2 tbsp demerara (raw brown) sugar

1 Preheat the oven to 200°C/400°F/Gas mark 6.

2 Put the pistachios, 4 tablespoons of the honey, the cinnamon and the orange juice and zest in a blender or food processor. Whiz together until the nuts are roughly chopped.

3 Unroll the pastry and lay it out on a baking tray that's big enough to fit the pastry. Spread the pistachio mixture over the pastry, leaving a 2cm (¾in) border around the edge.

4 Next, put the apricot halves, cut-side up, over the pistachio mixture and drizzle with the remaining honey.

5 Brush the beaten egg all around the 2cm (¾in) edge and sprinkle the demerara (raw brown) sugar over the top of the apricots and the 2cm (¾in) border.

6 Pop in the oven and bake for 15 minutes or until the pastry is risen and golden and the apricots have just softened.

7 Cut into slices and sprinkle with extra pistachios.

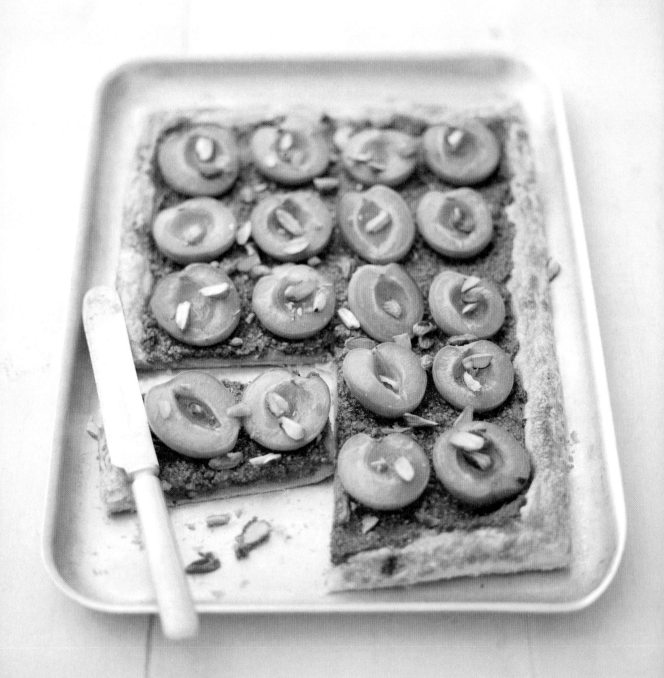

apricot and cherry crunchy oaty pudding

Use fresh fruit for this pud to get the full health benefit.

serves 6

900g (2lb) apricots, pitted
  and cut into large chunks

450g (1lb) cherries, pitted

2 tbsp demerara (raw
  brown) sugar

115g (4oz/1 cup) wholemeal
  (wholewheat) flour

25g (1oz/¼ cup) oats

25g (1oz/⅛ cups) sunflower
  seeds

50g (2oz/¼ cup) brown sugar

50g (2oz/¼ cup) unsalted
  butter, chilled and
  chopped into small pieces

low-fat crème fraîche,
  to serve

1 Preheat the oven to 190°C/375°F/Gas mark 5.

2 Put the apricot chunks in a 1.2 litre (2 pint/1.2 quart) ovenproof dish with the cherries and mix well. Sprinkle the demerara (raw brown) sugar over the top. Set aside.

3 Combine the flour, oats, sunflower seeds and brown sugar in a bowl. Add the butter chunks and rub the ingredients together using the tips of your fingers until the mixture resembles breadcrumbs (do not overmix). Sprinkle the oat mixture evenly over the fruit.

4 Bake for approximately 40 minutes or until the topping is golden brown and the syrup has started to bubble through the edges.

5 Serve while the pudding is still warm, with a dollop of crème fraîche.

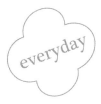

everyday

apple and pear sorbet

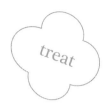
treat

This is an easy to make and refreshing dessert – perfect after a heavy meal.

serves 6

4 apples, peeled, cored
and chopped

4 pears, peeled, cored
and chopped

2 ready-to-eat dried
soft apricots

juice of 1 lemon

1 tsp ground cinnamon

4 tbsp caster
(superfine) sugar

1 Put the prepared apples and pears into a large lidded saucepan and add just enough water to cover the bottom of the pan. Cover the pan and simmer for 5–10 minutes until the fruit is soft. Set aside to cool.

2 Next, in a liquidiser or with a hand-held blender, purée the cooled apples and pears with the dried apricots, lemon juice and cinnamon.

3 Meanwhile, put the sugar into a small saucepan with 4 tablespoons of water and bring to the boil. Mix this syrup in with the fruit purée, then allow the mixture to cool completely.

4 Transfer to a freezerproof container and freeze for about 3 hours, stirring occasionally.

5 To serve, crush up with a fork and put into small glass bowls.

baked apples with cranberry and ginger

Simply divine!

serves 4

100g (3½oz/1 cup) fresh
   or frozen cranberries

2cm (¾in) fresh ginger,
   peeled and grated

2 tbsp demerara (raw
   brown) sugar

2 medium apples

150ml (5fl oz/⅔ cup)
   apple juice

4 tbsp low-fat or fat-free
   Greek yogurt, to serve

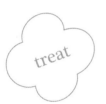

1 Preheat the oven to 180°C/350°F/Gas mark 4.

2 In a large bowl, mix the cranberries with the ginger
   and demerara sugar.

3 Slice the apples in half widthways and dig out the cores.
   Place the apples in a baking dish that's just big enough
   to support all the apple halves, but without too much
   spare room.

4 Pack the cranberry mixture into the hollows of the
   apples. Pour over the apple juice and bake in the oven
   for about 30 minutes or until the apples are soft, basting
   them with the apple juice halfway through.

5 Serve each apple half with some juice and a tablespoon
   of Greek yogurt.

filo apple and cinnamon tarts

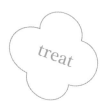
treat

This is a treat with sugar and a little butter – so be sure your main course is low on fat and salt … and go for a walk after eating!

serves 8

700g (1½lb) Bramley cooking apples

100g (3½oz/½ cup) light brown muscovado sugar

zest and juice of 2 lemons

½ tsp ground cinnamon, plus a good pinch extra, for dusting

50g (2oz/¼ cup) sultanas (golden raisins)

200g (7oz) shop-bought filo (phyllo) pastry

a little milk (to glue the pastry)

icing (confectioners') sugar, to dust

yogurt, to serve

1 Preheat the oven to 180°C/350°F/Gas mark 4.

2 Place the apples, muscovado sugar, lemon zest and juice, cinnamon and sultanas (golden raisins) in a large pan and cook gently for 5–7 minutes, stirring occasionally, until the apples have softened but still hold their shape. Allow to cool.

3 Unroll the pastry and cut into 32cm x 14cm (12½in x 5½in) squares, keeping the trimmings to one side. Take one of the squares and brush with a little milk, then place another square over the top at an angle to make a star shape. Repeat with 2 more squares of pastry, brushing each with milk, so each case is made up of 4 squares. Gently press the pastry into one of the holes in a standard 12-hole muffin tin. Repeat with the remaining pastry until you have 8 pastry cases.

4 Fill each case with the apple mixture, then brush the leftover trimmings with milk, scrunch them up and place on top of the tarts. Bake for 20–25 minutes until golden brown. Serve each tart dusted with icing (confectioners') sugar mixed with a good pinch of cinnamon, with a dollop of fat-free yogurt if you fancy.

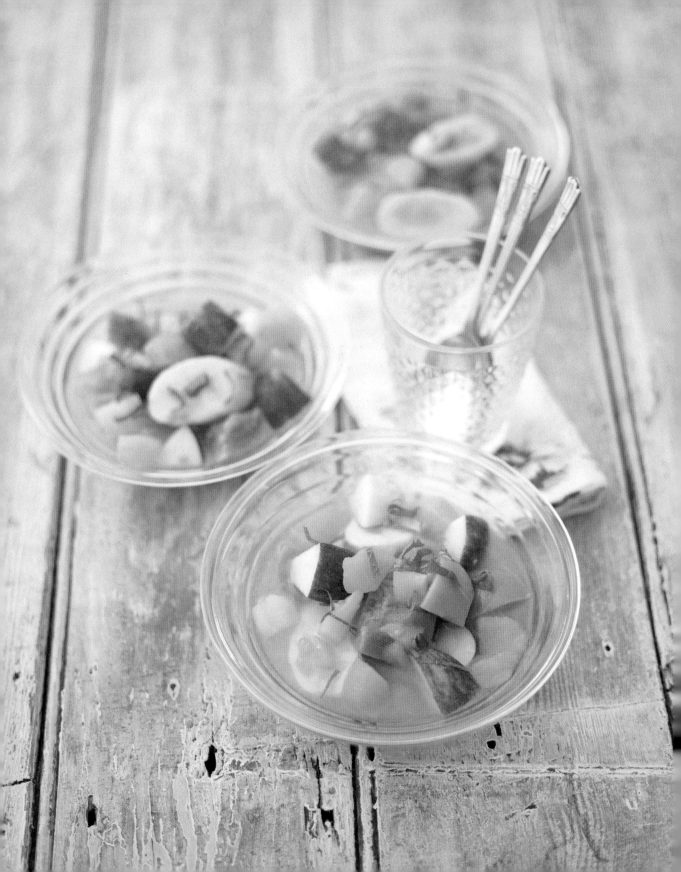

sweet-and-sour fruit salad

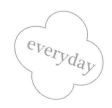

everyday

An everyday classic is given a twist with some exotic tastes. This mixture of fresh and canned fruit, which has a sweet-and-sour flavour, is very cooling, especially in the summer months. You can serve tea or fresh fruit juice with this dish.

serves 4

400g (14oz) tinned mixed
  fruit cocktail

400g (14oz) tinned guavas
  in natural juice

2 large bananas

3 apples

2 tbsp lemon juice

½ tsp ground ginger

shredded fresh mint,
  to decorate

yogurt, to serve

1 Drain the fruit cocktail and place the fruit in a deep bowl. Mix in the guavas and their juice.

2 Peel the bananas and cut them into slices.

3 Wash the apples. Don't peel them, but do core them, then cut them into dice. Add the fresh fruit to the bowl and mix in the tinned fruit. Finally, add the lemon juice and ginger and stir in well.

4 Transfer to a serving bowl and decorate with a shredded few fresh mint leaves. Serve on its own or with low-fat thick yogurt.

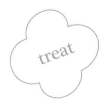
treat

chocolate vanilla mousse

This recipe was very kindly donated to me by the Chocolate Lady Extraordinaire, Claire Burnet of Chococo, the makers of beautiful handmade chocolates. It's definitely a treat but, still, without any additional dairy. Enjoy it every now and again.

serves 4

200g (7oz) good-quality dark chocolate (ideally with 70 per cent cocoa solids) or 150g (5oz) dark chocolate and 50g (2oz) milk chocolate*

1 tsp vanilla essence (extract)

to serve

cocoa powder, for dusting

crème fraîche, berries or biscotti (optional)

* Including a little milk chocolate (with a minimum of 35 per cent cocoa solids) just takes the edge off the intensity of pure dark chocolate. Mousses made with just dark chocolate will set firmer than those made with the inclusion of milk chocolate.

1 Chop the chocolate into small chunks and place in a heatproof glass bowl set over a pan of barely simmering water. Melt the chocolate gently. Ensure that the water in the pan does not touch the bottom of the bowl.

2 Once the chocolate is melted, add 200ml (7fl oz/¾ cup) of just-boiled water (do not add the water while it is still boiling, as it may scorch the chocolate) in three equal lots, stirring after each addition to form a smooth but quite runny mixture.

3 Add the vanilla essence (extract) to the mixture and blend in. The mixture is very runny at this point but don't worry – it will thicken as it cools.

4 Pour the mixture into a lipped jug (pitcher), then pour it into small coffee cups or glasses. (Using a lipped jug (pitcher) allows you to fill the cups easily without it dripping everywhere.) These mousses are rich, so you don't want big portions.

Tip:
Any chocolate used must be made with pure cocoa butter and contain no added vegetable fats. Any such ingredients have to be declared on chocolate packaging, so can be easily avoided.

5 Put the mousses into the refrigerator to set for at least 1 hour, but bring back to room temperature before serving so they soften to the right consistency.

6 To serve, dust with cocoa powder and serve as they are, or with a dollop of crème fraîche, fresh berries or a crunchy biscotti-type biscuit.

Flavour variation

Make a tea infusion by adding a dessertspoonful of aromatic loose leaf tea such as Lapsang souchong, Moroccan mint or Earl Grey to 200ml (7fl oz/¾ cup) boiling water. Allow to infuse for 2 minutes, then strain the tea and add this to the melted chocolate in place of the just-boiled water.

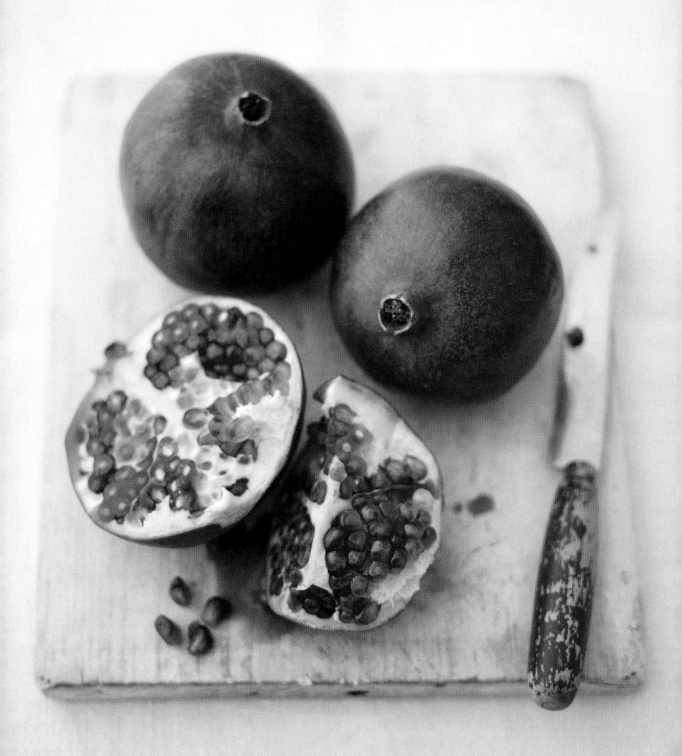

drinks

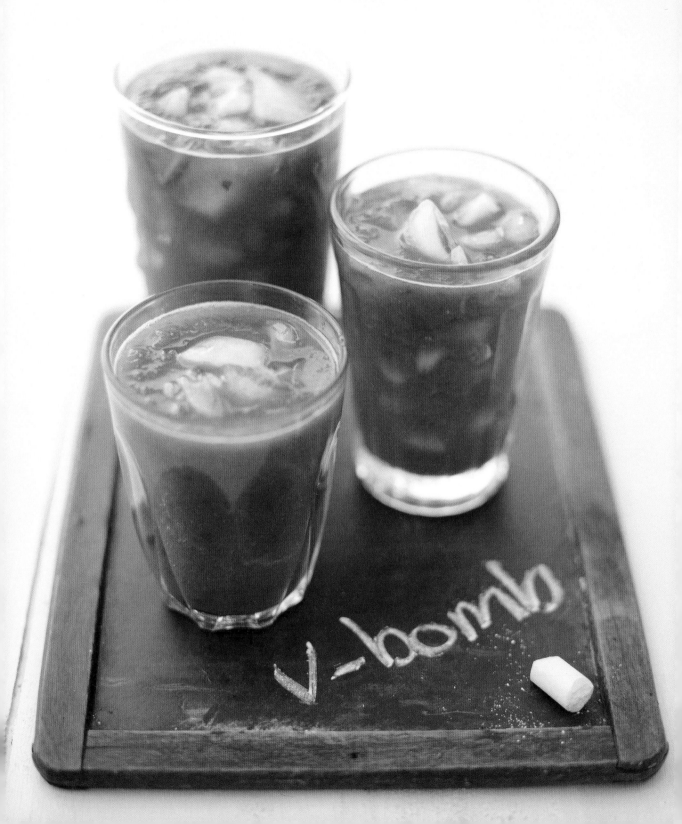

vitamin bomb drink

everyday

Speaks for itself!

serves 4

1 green (bell) pepper, deseeded and sliced

1 red (bell) pepper, deseeded and sliced

½ cucumber, sliced

1 onion, peeled and cut into chunks

2 tbsp lemon juice

1 garlic clove, peeled

cayenne pepper, to taste

600ml (1 pint/2½ cups) tomato juice

ice cubes, to serve

1 Put all the ingredients except the tomato juice into a blender and blitz it until well mixed and smooth. Then pour in the tomato juice and blend for another 30 seconds.

2 Serve the drink on ice.

elly's mum's joint-care drink

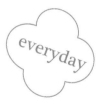
everyday

My friend Elly's mum swears by this drink. She takes it every day and, recently, after some joint problems, I've started to take it, too. Whether it works or not, I'm not sure, but it's a lovely drink that makes a healthy alternative to tea or coffee. Simply mix with 250ml (9fl oz/1 cup) boiling water and drink.

serves 1

1 tsp organic honey

1 tbsp apple cider vinegar

Along with a lot of other 'old wives tales', my Grandma used to say 'An apple a day keeps the doctor away'. Actually, many of these old sayings came from a sensible source. Apples are the central ingredient in apple cider vinegar and it is proven to give a host of health benefits. High in potassium and magnesium, apple cider vinegar is thought to help with joints, tissues, digestion and blood pressure. You see, your grandma did know what she was talking about!

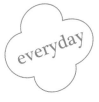

carrot & apple smoothie

A drink that slides down particularly well! This recipe shows a slightly unusual approach to making a smoothie, but it's totally worth the effort.

serves 2

3 medium carrots, peeled
  and sliced

175ml (6 fl oz/¾ cup)
  boiling water

375ml (13fl oz/1½ cups)
  apple juice

1 In a small lidded saucepan set over a medium heat, cook the carrots in the boiling water for about 20 minutes or until very tender. Allow the carrots to cool in the water.

2 Transfer the carrots and cooking liquid to blender or liquidiser, add the apple juice and blitz until smooth. Feel free to add a little more apple juice to get your desired consistency.

tangy tomato mocktail

Sweet, yet tangy, this drink makes an excellent alcohol-free alternative to a cocktail – it is guilt free and packed with vitamin C. Be sure to use very ripe fruit for the best results.

serves 4

1 ripe mango, peeled and
  roughly chopped

500g (1lb 2oz) vine
  tomatoes, peeled and
  roughly chopped

575g (1lb 5oz) watermelon,
  peeled and roughly
  chopped

zest and juice of 1 orange

zest and juice of 1 lime

5–6 ice cubes

1 Simply put all the prepared ingredients into a food processor and blend together with the ice cubes to make a thick slush. Serve immediately.

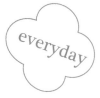

tart cocktail

treat

The rhubarb in this nectar gives a delicious tartness. Adding a little hint of mint gives it another dimension and takes off the edge of the tartness. Drinking this cocktail is an experience you'll want to repeat!

serves 4

450g (1lb) rhubarb, cut into 5cm (2in) lengths

5 tbsp caster (superfine) sugar

2 tbsp lemon juice

1 small handful of fresh mint leaves, plus sprigs of mint, to garnish

600ml (1 pint/2½ cups) sparkling mineral water

1 Put the rhubarb, sugar, lemon juice, mint and 350ml (12fl oz/1½ cups) of water in a large saucepan set over a medium heat. Bring to the boil, then reduce the heat and simmer, uncovered, for 5 minutes or until the rhubarb begins to collapse. Remove from the heat and leave to cool for about an hour.

2 Strain out and discard the rhubarb and the mint leaves. Chill the rhubarb liquid in the refrigerator before serving.

3 When ready to serve, combine equal amounts of rhubarb liquid and sparkling mineral water in each glass and add a sprig of mint and a couple of ice cubes.

pineapple & strawberry smoothie

everyday

Drinking smoothies is one of the best ways of filling up on fruit, and therefore, nutrients and energy. Try this one out on the kids – it's fully flavour-loaded, and so good for them.

serves 2

225g (8oz/1½ cups) strawberries

225ml (8fl oz/1 cup) unsweetened pineapple juice

150g (5oz/⅔ cup) low-fat strawberry yogurt

1 Put all the ingredients into a smoothie maker or blender and whiz up until smooth. Serve immediately. Try to serve this straight away, before the fruit changes colour, but it will store in the refrigerator for up to 12 hours (just give it a good stir before serving).

cranberry and pomegranate sparkler

Cranberries and pomegranates contain antioxidants that will boost your immunity as cold and flu season rolls around. This refreshing glassful offers a tasty and healthy way to rehydrate.

serves 4

250ml (9fl oz/1 cup) cranberry juice

250ml (9fl oz/1 cup) pomegranate juice

250ml (9fl oz/1 cup) sparkling mineral water

juice of ½ lime

2 slices of lime

1 Divide the ingredients (except the lime slices) equally between 2 tall glasses. Stir, add ice, and serve with a slice of lime.

spiced grape juicy lucy

This Juicy Lucy is perfect when served warm, but translates to a refreshing cold drink easily – just cool, refrigerate and add lots of crushed ice just before serving.

serves 2

425ml (15fl oz/1¾ cups) red grape juice

zest and juice of 1 large orange

pinch of ground allspice

12 green cardamom pods, lightly crushed

1 cinnamon stick

6 cloves

1 tbsp clear honey

crushed ice, to serve (if serving cold)

1 Combine all the ingredients in a large saucepan and simmer over a medium heat for 5 minutes, then reduce the heat to low and continue simmering for 10 minutes.

2 Remove from the heat and leave to cool for 1 hour, then serve with crushed ice.

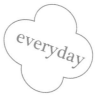

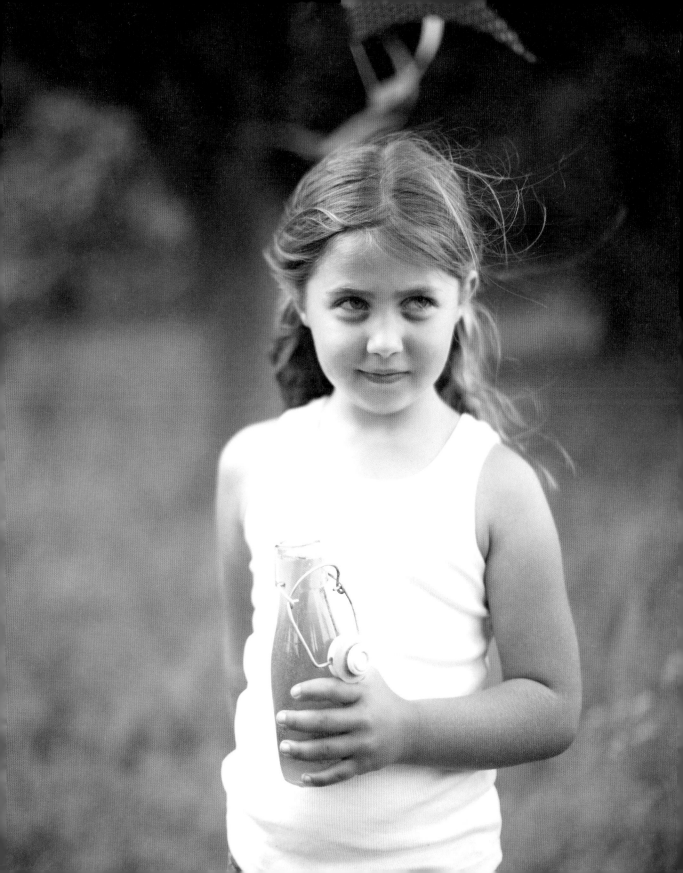

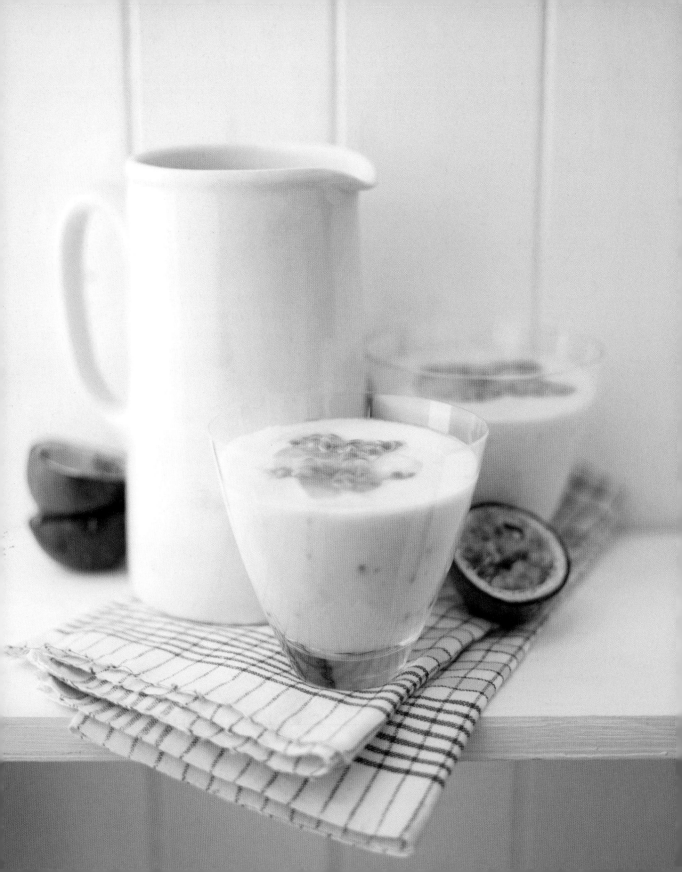

passion fruit and banana smoothie

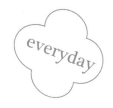

everyday

My family are passionate about this drink. Smoothies made with bananas don't keep too well, which used to worry me, but actually we never have any of this super smoothie left over!

serves 4

4 ripe passion fruits

4 ripe bananas, peeled and chopped

225g (8oz) seedless red or white grapes

150g (5oz/⅔ cup) low-fat bio-yogurt

½ tsp vanilla essence (extract)

8 ice cubes

1 Cut the passion fruits in half and scoop out the pulp. Reserve 1 tablespoon of the pulp to decorate your smoothies.

2 Put the rest of the pulp, along with all the other ingredients, into a smoothie maker or blender and whiz up until smooth. Serve with the extra pulp drizzled on top. If the smoothie is a little too thick for your liking, add a tablespoon or 2 of skimmed (skim) milk, stirred in just before serving.

cherry and berry smoothie

Vibrant colours, vibrant flavours and all to give you some vibrant energy!

serves 2

200g (7oz/1⅓ cups) strawberries, hulled

200g (7oz/1⅓ cups) fresh or frozen pitted dark sweet cherries

200g (7oz/1⅔ cups) raspberries

250ml (9fl oz/1 cup) pomegranate juice, chilled

200g (7oz/1⅓ cups) blueberries

1 Wash all the fruit, put it into a blender with the juice and whiz up. Drink straight away.

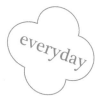

everyday

index

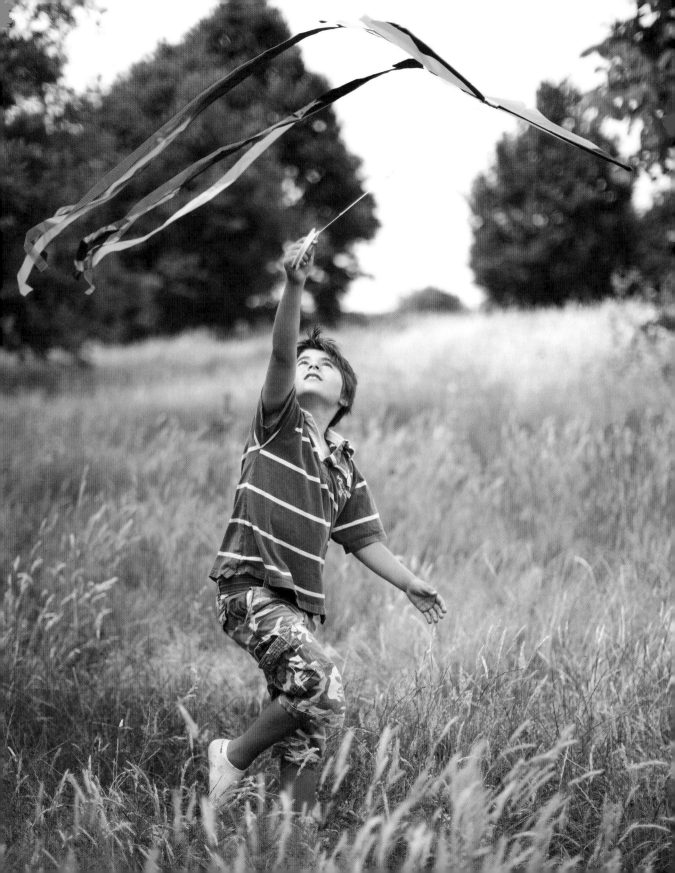

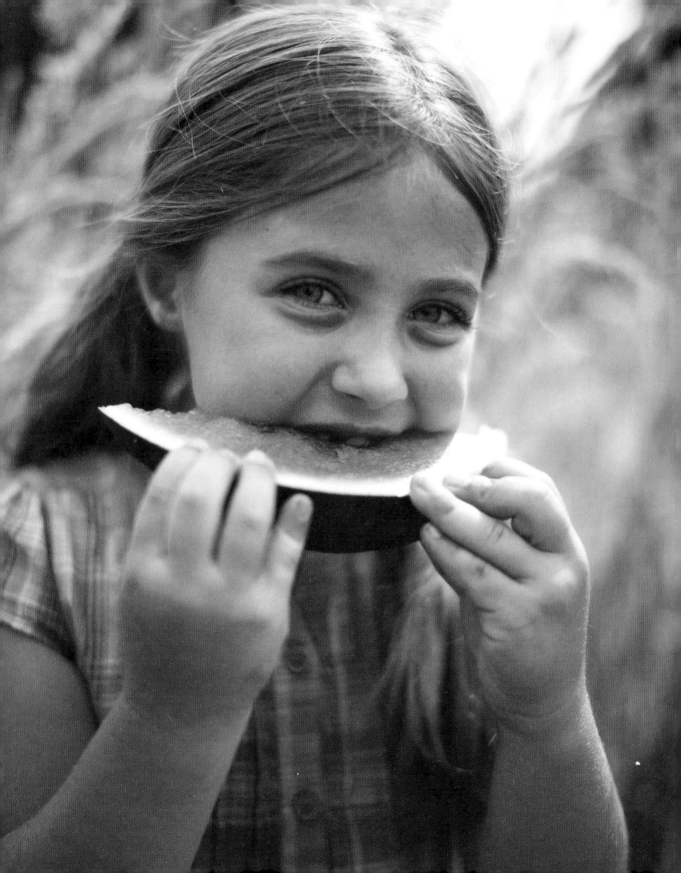

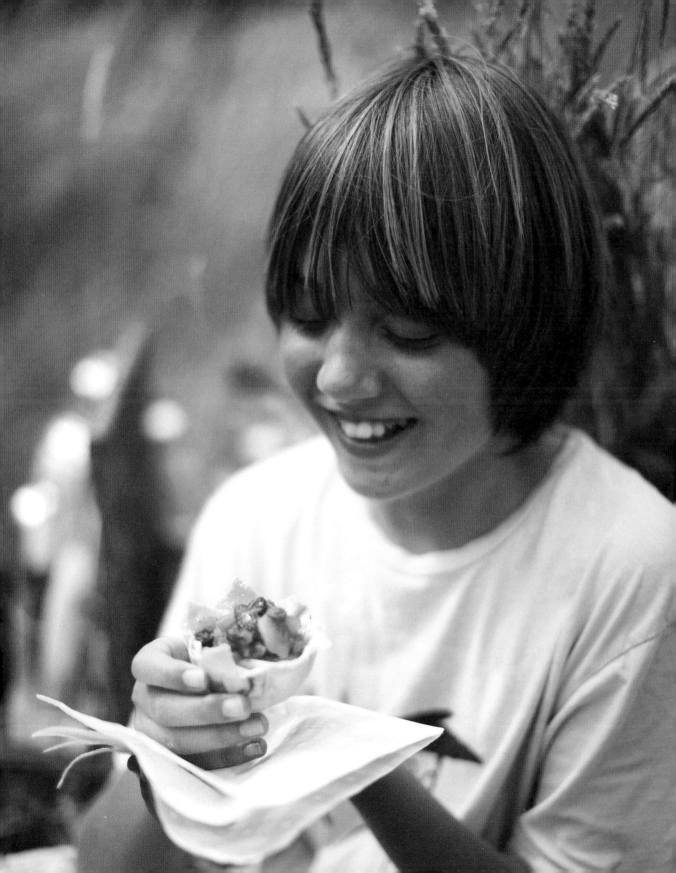

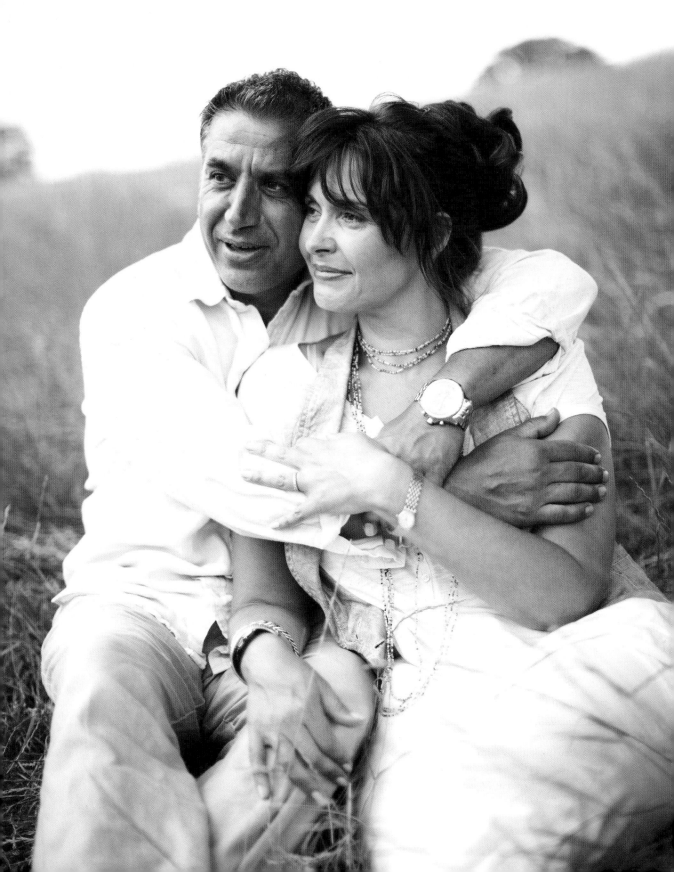

acknowledgements

I give my sincere thanks to everyone who has helped me with the production of my book. To Clare Hulton, my literary agent, who makes a wonderful sounding board for my zillions of ideas. Thank you to Jenny Heller, Lizzy Gray, Helen Hawksfield, Salima Hirani, Heike Schuessler, Sophie Martin and the rest of the team at the wonderful, brilliant and supportive HarperCollins. Thank you also to Myles New for taking such amazing pictures and making my hair look better and to Lorna Brash for paying such kind detail to my recipes for the photographs. My family are always a wonderful help to me, especially Tarik, Kazim and Lela. You are my most honest critics so thank you – I think!

Keep updated by visiting www.sally-bee.com